WRAPPED IN *Love*

WRAPPED IN *Love*

Soft and Snugly Prayer Shawls for Children

SYLVIA SCOTT

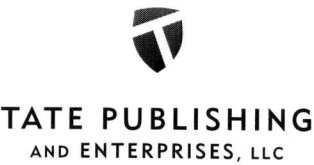

TATE PUBLISHING
AND ENTERPRISES, LLC

Wrapped In Love
Copyright © 2012 by Sylvia Scott. All rights reserved.

No part of this publication may be reproduced, stored in a retrieval system or transmitted in any way by any means, electronic, mechanical, photocopy, recording or otherwise without the prior permission of the author except as provided by USA copyright law.

The opinions expressed by the author are not necessarily those of Tate Publishing, LLC.

Published by Tate Publishing & Enterprises, LLC
127 E. Trade Center Terrace | Mustang, Oklahoma 73064 USA
1.888.361.9473 | www.tatepublishing.com

Tate Publishing is committed to excellence in the publishing industry. The company reflects the philosophy established by the founders, based on Psalm 68:11,
"The Lord gave the word and great was the company of those who published it."

Book design copyright © 2012 by Tate Publishing, LLC. All rights reserved.
Cover design by Kenna Davis
Interior design by Chelsea Womble

Published in the United States of America

ISBN: 978-1-61862-272-3
1. Crafts & Hobbies / Needlework / Knitting
2. Religion / Christian Ministry / Children
12.03.08

Dedicated to Helen Larsen, my confidant, my mentor, and my friend, in whose presence I always felt wrapped in love. She went to be with the Lord on August 28, 2011.

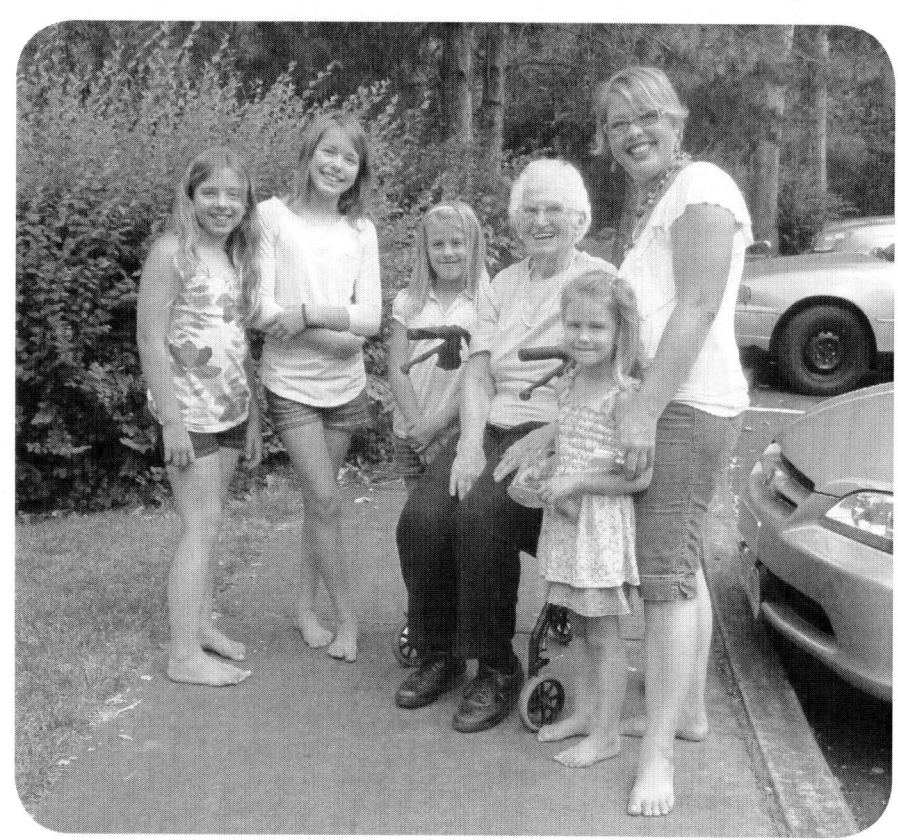

And to my sister, Eleanor, who taught me many things, including how to knit.

TABLE OF CONTENTS

INTRODUCTION 9
GENESIS OF THE SOFT AND SNUGLY PRAYER SHAWLS FOR CHILDREN 11
DIRECTIONS FOR THE DOUBLE-KNITTING TECHNIQUE 13
PHOTOS OF PATTERNS 17

PATTERNS:

Happy Faces 34
Heart Happy Faces 35
Ascending Hearts 36
Teddy Bears 37
Two Sports Balls 38
Skateboards 39
Downhill Bicycles 40
Let's Play Football 41
Acoustic Guitar 42
Electric Bass Guitar 44
Come Fly with Me 46
Quiet Sailboats 47
Beautiful Butterflies 48
Ducks in a Row 49
Scottie Dogs 50
Angels 51

INTRODUCTION

Hand crafted shawls have been offering comfort and blessing for generations. They are a tangible bond connecting the giver and the recipient to each other and to the Lord who sends the blessings.

Currently churches everywhere are participating in prayer shawl ministries. This movement is led, primarily, by Janet Bristow and Victoria A. Cole-Galo, founders of shawlministry.com. Their website or their book *The Prayer Shawl Companion,* will give you everything you need to begin, or enhance a prayer shawl ministry in your church.

Wrapped in Love: Soft and Snugly Prayer Shawls for Children will enrich your existing prayer shawl ministry. It offers sixteen enchanting patterns designed to capture the attention of children, to remind them that they are loved and cared for, and to give them something tangible to wrap up in when they are concerned. Also included is a pattern for a mini-shawl in which the child can wrap their doll, teddy bear, or even their action toy. When comforting a toy, the child can project their own trauma and become the comforter.

GENESIS OF THE SOFT AND SNUGLY PRAYER SHAWLS FOR CHILDREN

One day, a member of our very active prayer shawl ministry delivered a shawl to a lady with stage-four breast cancer. Her four little girls watched as she unwrapped the shawl.

Knowing that she had already been given a shawl from another church, one of the girls asked her mother, "What will we do if we get any more shawls?"

To which the mother replied, "We'll just wrap up in them and pray."

It was immediately decided that each girl should have her own shawl created in little girl colors. (See front cover.)

Today, the mother is in remission and is, in fact, homeschooling her girls.

In the mother's words:

> When I was diagnosed with cancer, I knew, in the very depth of my soul, that I do not worship a God who capriciously inflicts diseases on mothers with young children. I worship a God who straddles the incomprehensibility of grace and truth, who defies definition or boundary, who is most present when we choose to serve one another, in whatever way we find. The church prayer shawl ministry mentioned above fulfilled that most-essential mandate of Christ: "What you've done unto the least of these, you've done unto me." The shawls designed for and delivered to my daughters acknowledged their own devastation. My diagnosis was, in every sense, our shared tragedy. The shawls, intended especially for them, fulfilled one of Jesus' primary mandates: "Suffer the little children to come unto me."
>
> While I am enjoying an extended, much hoped-for and gratitude-filled remission, I will not forget those who gave to my family without requiring me to do the thinking for them; rather, they saw a need and filled it. Such innovative, generous giving is the heart of Christian service. No lip service, only action. May we all embrace this same spirit of service.

My prayer is that the patterns in this book will assist you in bringing comfort to children, and that they will not only feel wrapped in a shawl but will feel wrapped in Christ's love as well.

DIRECTIONS FOR THE DOUBLE-KNITTING TECHNIQUE

Materials:

- Two 6 oz. skeins of Caron Simply Soft® yarn (one skein of each color) There is enough yarn in these two skeins to make a shawl and a mini-shawl, including the fringe for each.
- Size 13 knitting needles
- Crochet hook for attaching fringe

Abbreviations:

K – knit

P – purl

CO – cast on

BO – bind off

Double knitting is a technique using two colors of yarn at the same time. The knit stitches form the color on the front while the contrasting purl stitches show on the back. When working the second row, the colors are reversed. The knit stitches will be worked in the contrasting color, and the purl stitches will show on the front in the first color. Each pattern square represents 2 stitches, the knit followed by the contrasting purl. Work the chart from right to left on the front side and from left to right on the back side.

When I am counting the pattern, I say, "One and two and three and four and," etc. The number representing the knit stitch, and the "and" representing the contrasting purl stitch. I also like to start row 1 with the darker color. That helps as I work up the pattern to remember that all odd numbered rows show the darker color as background when following the pattern from right to left, and the even numbered rows show the lighter color when following the pattern from left to right.

WRAPPED IN LOVE

Before starting a shawl, it is best to learn the double knitting technique by making a mini-shawl. This will give you practice in making the double knit stitches, as well as practice with a simple pattern.

CO 30 stitches (15 of each color) using the alternating two-color long tail cast on method. (Demonstrations for this procedure are easily found on the Internet. Google: alternating two-color long tail cast-on.) Leave an eight-inch "tail" of each strand of yarn. End the cast on with the darker color so when you begin row one with K1, the first color on the needle will be the darker color. Then move both strands to the front and P1 with the contrasting lighter color. Continue K1 and P1 across the row, always moving both strands to the back or front before each stitch, and using the same color yarn as the next stitch on the needle. To maintain the proper tension, when inserting the needle in the purl stitch, pull each strand of yarn tight. In row two, follow the design established on row one. Knit in the color of the knit stitch on the needle, move both yarns to the front, and purl in the color of the purl stitch on the needle. Continue across the row, alternating K1 and P1. All of the patterns start with a few rows of background before beginning the pattern. This will give you a chance to observe the two sides of the fabric making a different solid color on each side before you start the pattern.

As you start each row, be sure to wrap the knit yarn under and around the purl yarn. This gives a nice, tight edge to the shawl.

By the end of a row or two, it will be obvious that the yarn is twisting. This is necessary to achieve the soft, one-piece double-knit fabric.

To accommodate this, stop knitting and follow these directions:

1. Put both skeins of yarn in a plastic grocery bag.

2. Pull out about 6-10 yards of both colors. (As you work with this procedure, you will learn how much length is comfortable for you.)

3. Wrap the yarn once or twice around each individual handle of the bag, and tie the handles together tightly enough so that the yarn does not slip out of the bag.

4. Now, take hold of the two strands of yarn about 2 1/2 feet from the bag. Lift the bag so it hangs free, and holding the bag away from your body with one hand, spin the bag in a clockwise direction with the other hand until it won't twist any more. At this point, let go of the two strands of yarn, lift the bag up to allow the twists to move toward the needles, loosening the tension on the twists. Repeat this procedure two or three times more.

5. Lift the bag up again so the twists equalize along the two strands of yarn. Don't allow the twist to get too tight close to the needles. Untie the bag and:

Mini-Shawl (approx. 5"X 18")

6. Put the loosely twisted yarn back in the plastic bag and continue knitting. Now, as you begin to knit, the natural twist will loosen rather than tighten, making the double-knit process possible. After a few rows, the twist will be gone. Simply repeat steps 1-6 and continue knitting.

Note: When the shawl is about half done, add some weight to the bag to make the spinning easier.

Continue the mini-shawl pattern until finished. Follow the directions for the fringe, using a 3-inch cardboard or a deck of cards. You will only need 60 strands of fringe to complete both ends of the mini-shawl. Now you have learned how to do the double knitting technique, follow the pattern and twist the yarn. You have also created a small shawl that a child can use to comfort their doll, stuffed animal, or even an action figure.

Next select a pattern and the colors you will use to make it.

To begin the shawl, cast on 80 stitches using the alternating 2-color long tail cast-on. Continue to work the number of rows at the bottom of the pattern that are blank. When beginning the pattern, indicated by the shaded dots, remember to read it from right to left when working the front of the shawl, and from left to right when working the back side. To check your work, count the stitches as you would any pattern, counting only the knit stitches. Both sides of the pattern will emerge at the same time. When you have reached the top of the pattern chart, continue working from top to bottom to create the second half of the shawl. Finish by binding off with the knit stitches as to knit and the purl stitches as to purl, using the matching color for each stitch. Leave a "tail" to be used as fringe. There are no ends to be woven in on the shawl.

Fringe:

Cut a piece of corrugated cardboard 6" by 6," or use a CD cover or book of the same size. Wrap both colors of yarn round the cardboard 10 times (20 strands). Cut the yarn on one edge. Tie individual knots about 1" from each of the ends. Repeat this process 7 more times until you have 160 strands, with knots near the end of each piece.

Now, using a crochet hook, draw the middle of a matching colored strand through the end of each row of ribbing. Pull the ends of the strands through the loop and tighten. Continue across both ends of the shawl. The "tails" left from casting on and binding off will become part of the fringe.

Happy Faces

This was the first children's shawl that I made. These shawls can be created in any colors you choose. As noted, the ones for the four little girls were all done in pink, with a contrasting pastel color. The one pictured here in blue and yellow was given the first time we had a need for a boy shawl. Children quickly relate to the bright, smiley faces and feel the comfort of being wrapped in them.

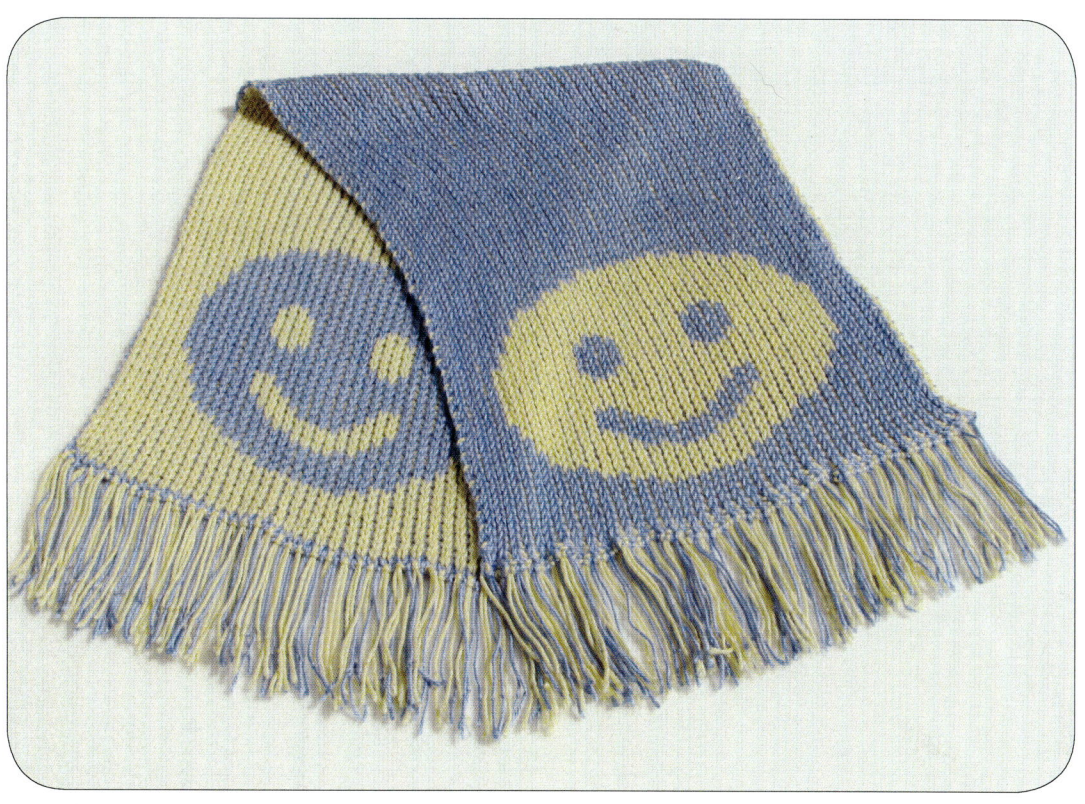

Heart Happy Faces

A variation of the happy face is the heart happy face. It adds a dimension of love while still giving the child the feeling of being wrapped in something with personality.

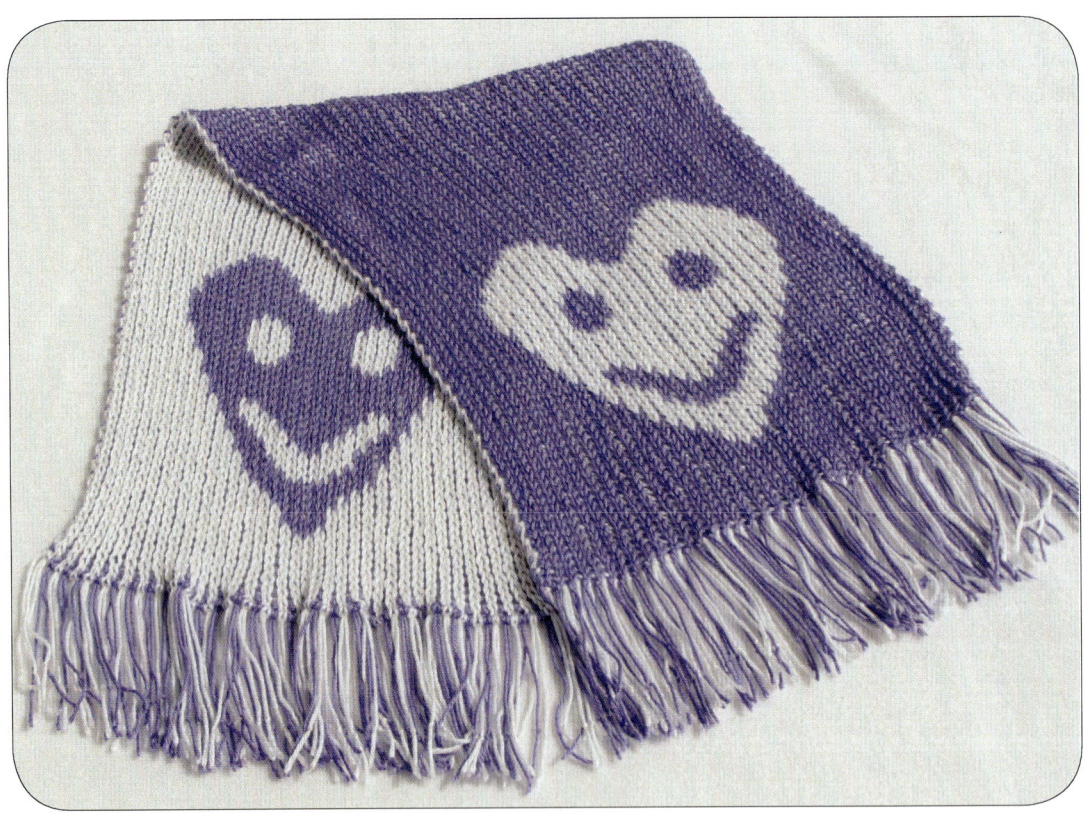

Ascending Hearts

Perhaps a slightly older child would like the ascending hearts, which appear to float up and around the shoulders.

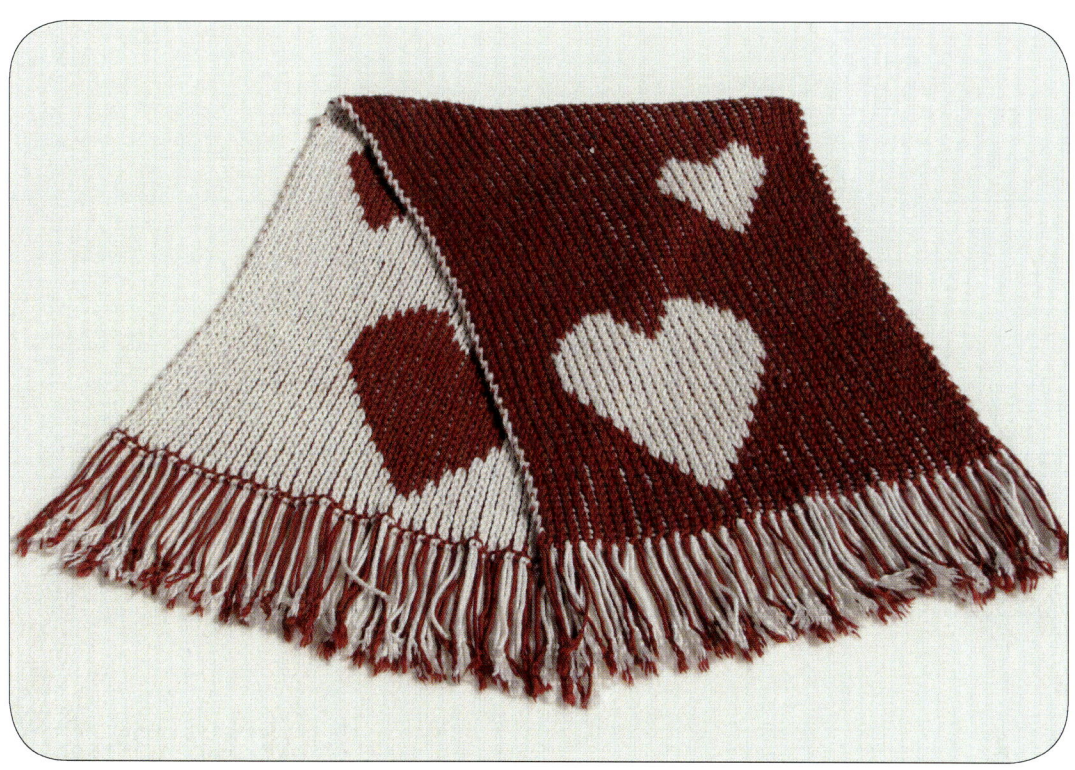

Teddy Bears

Teddy bears are universally loved by both boys and girls of all ages. This one, with his bright eyes and happy face, will be a favorite of all children. When knitted in baby colors and without fringe, this pattern makes an ideal gift for a newborn.

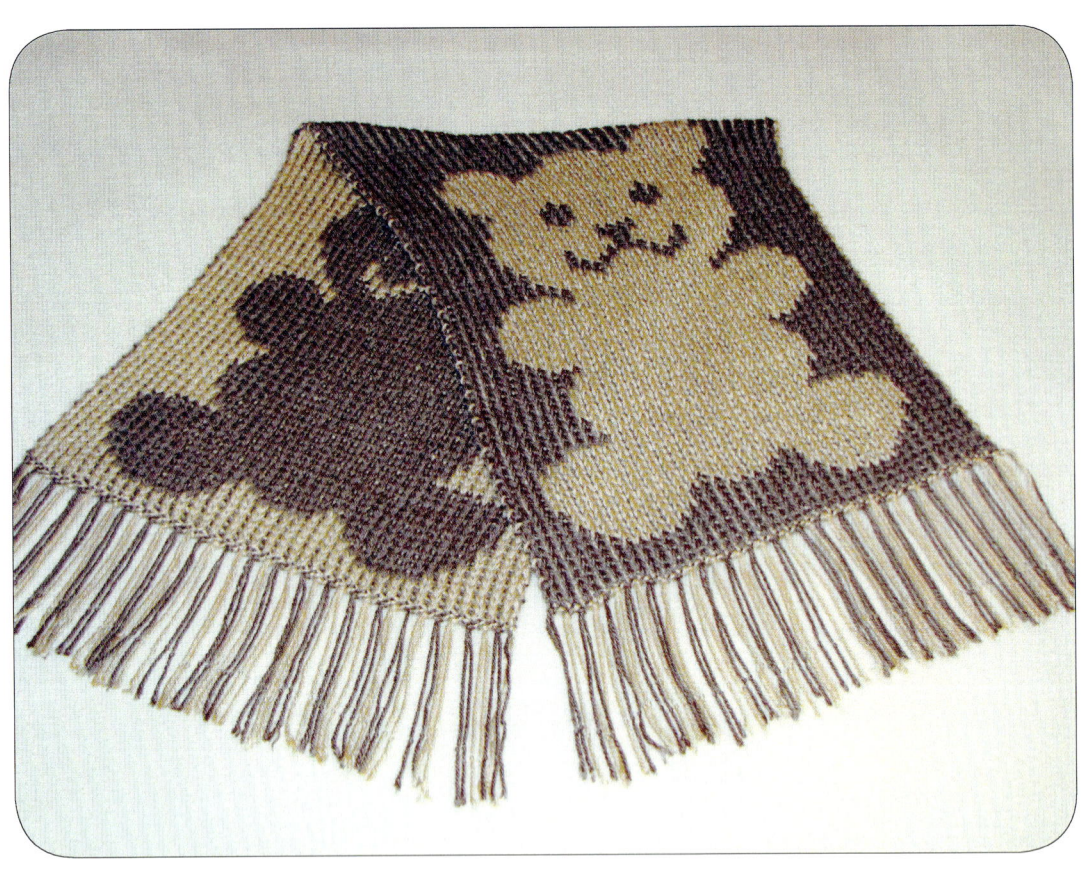

Two Sports Balls

Both girls and boys like sports. These balls were created to look like a basketball and a volleyball. The shawl is created in brown and white and can be left to look like a basketball and a volleyball. However, after the shawl is completed, if desired, lines can be chain-stitched to make the white ball resemble a soccer ball.

Just for fun, the background was reversed at the midpoint so that both balls would show when the shawl is wrapped around the shoulders.

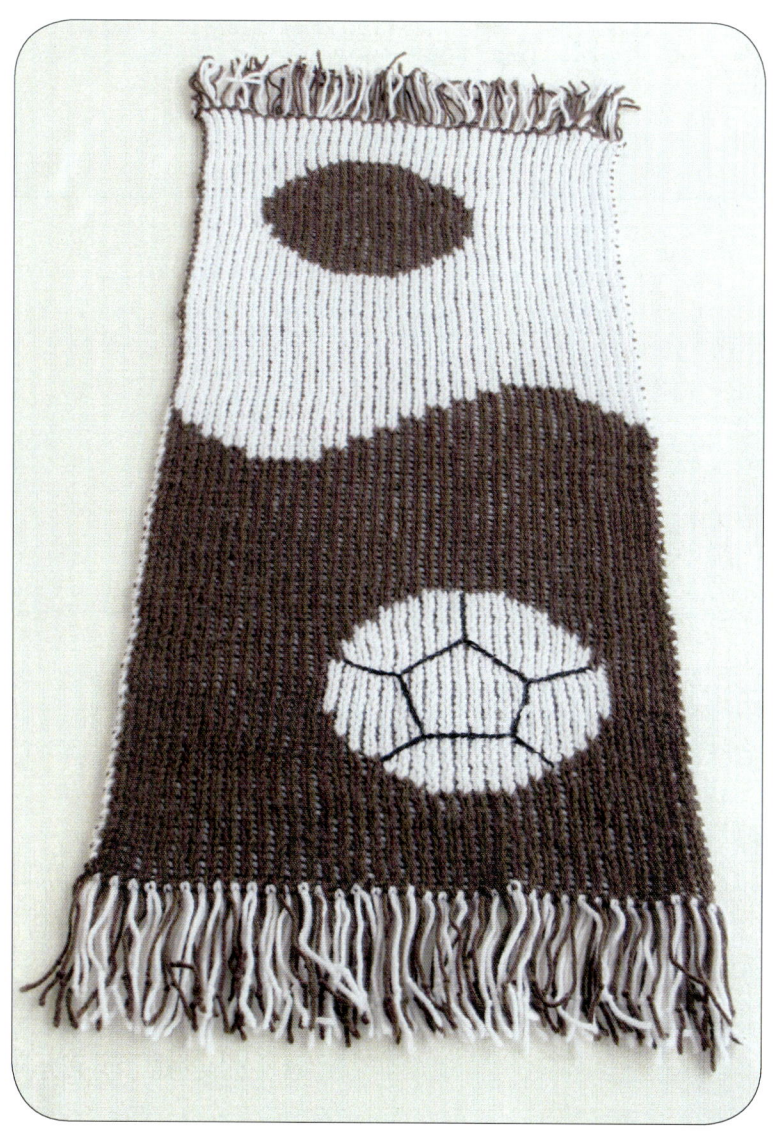

Skateboards

What could be more fun for older children, 'tweens, or even teens than a skateboard? It appears to be ready for someone to hop aboard and ride away. This one will be a real favorite. Try it in a variety of bright colors.

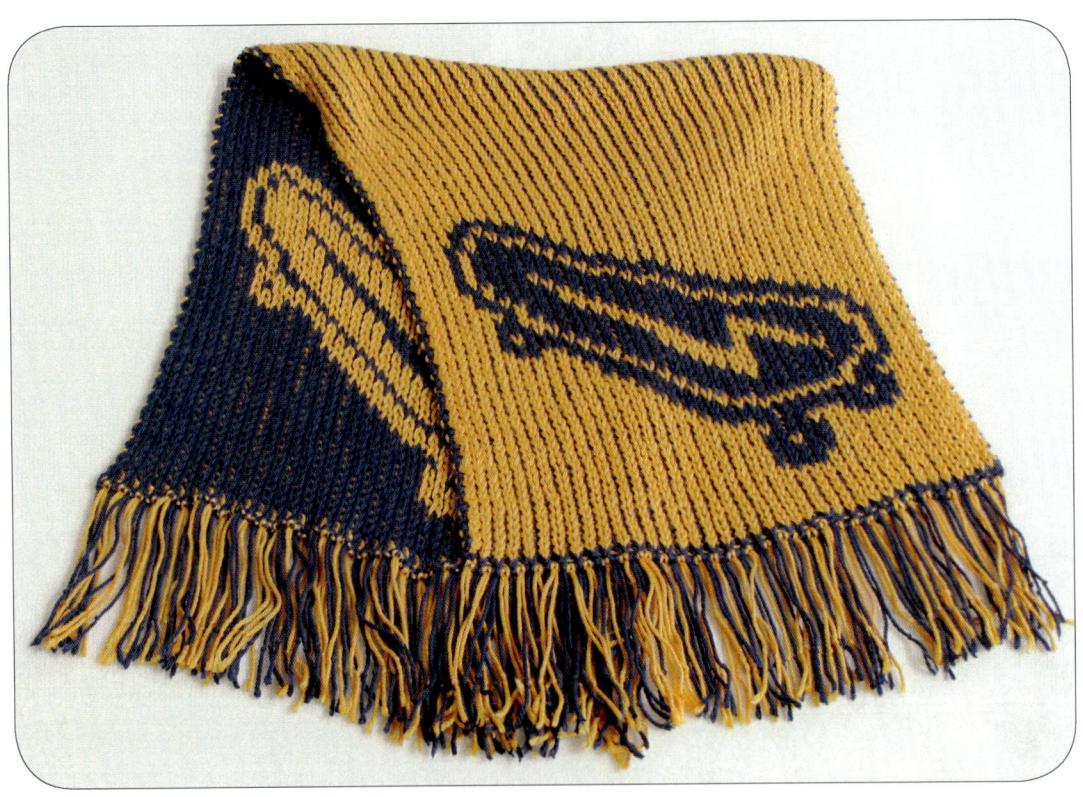

Downhill Bicycles

Whipping downhill on a bicycle may be just the answer for a child who is in need of a diversion.

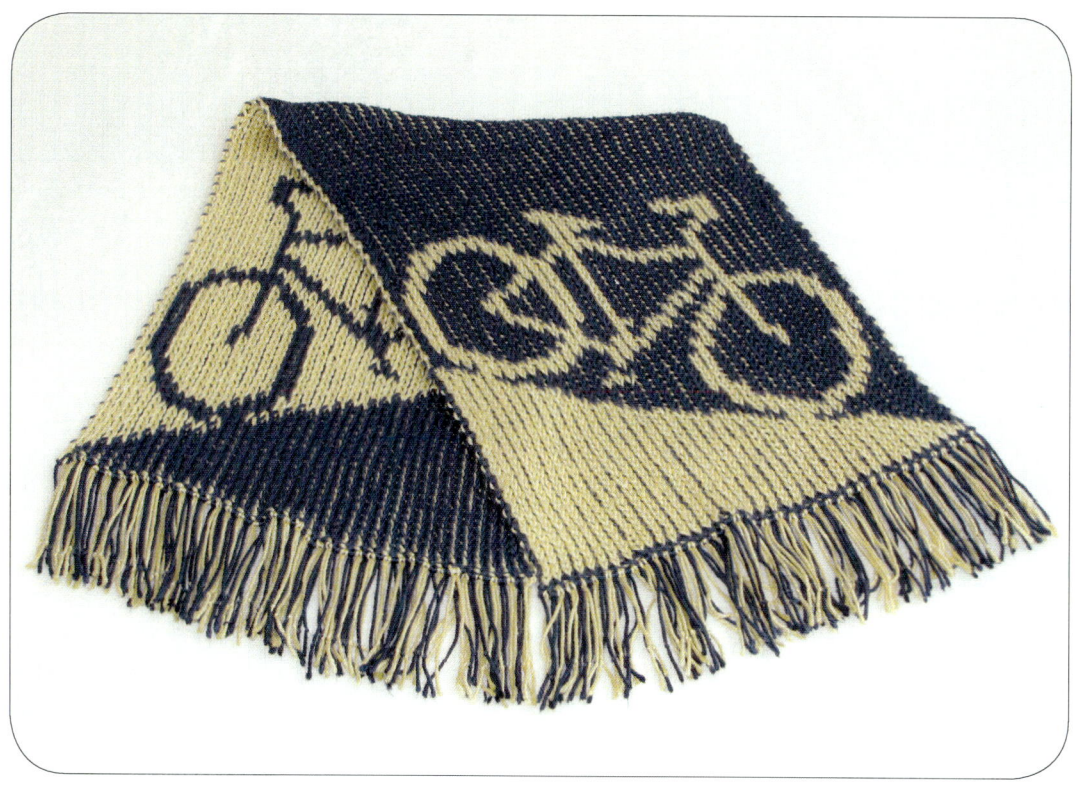

Let's Play Football

Feeling like a touchdown, or at least a field goal, is possible, this football shawl will put the child right on the playing field. Here's an idea! Try knitting this one in the team colors of the child's favorite football team.

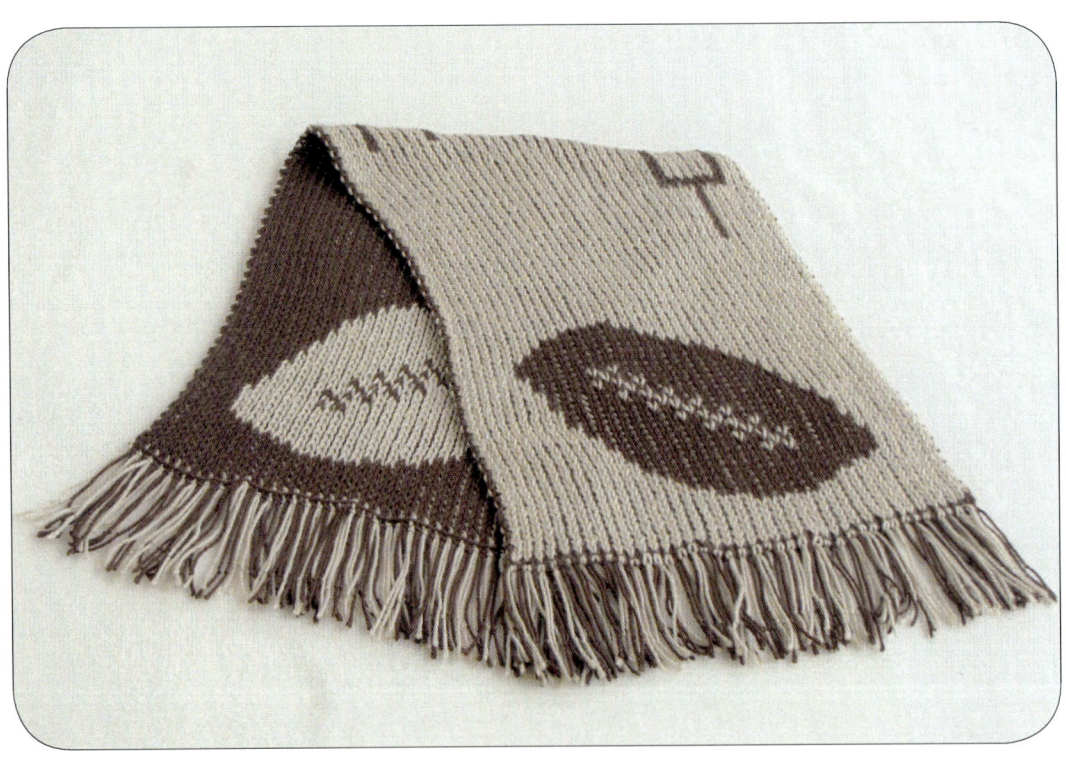

Acoustic Guitar

Is there a child who would not like to be completely wrapped up in a guitar?

The strings are made by embroidering them up the six rows and then attaching them to the knobs at the top, leaving the ends loose as they are on a real guitar.

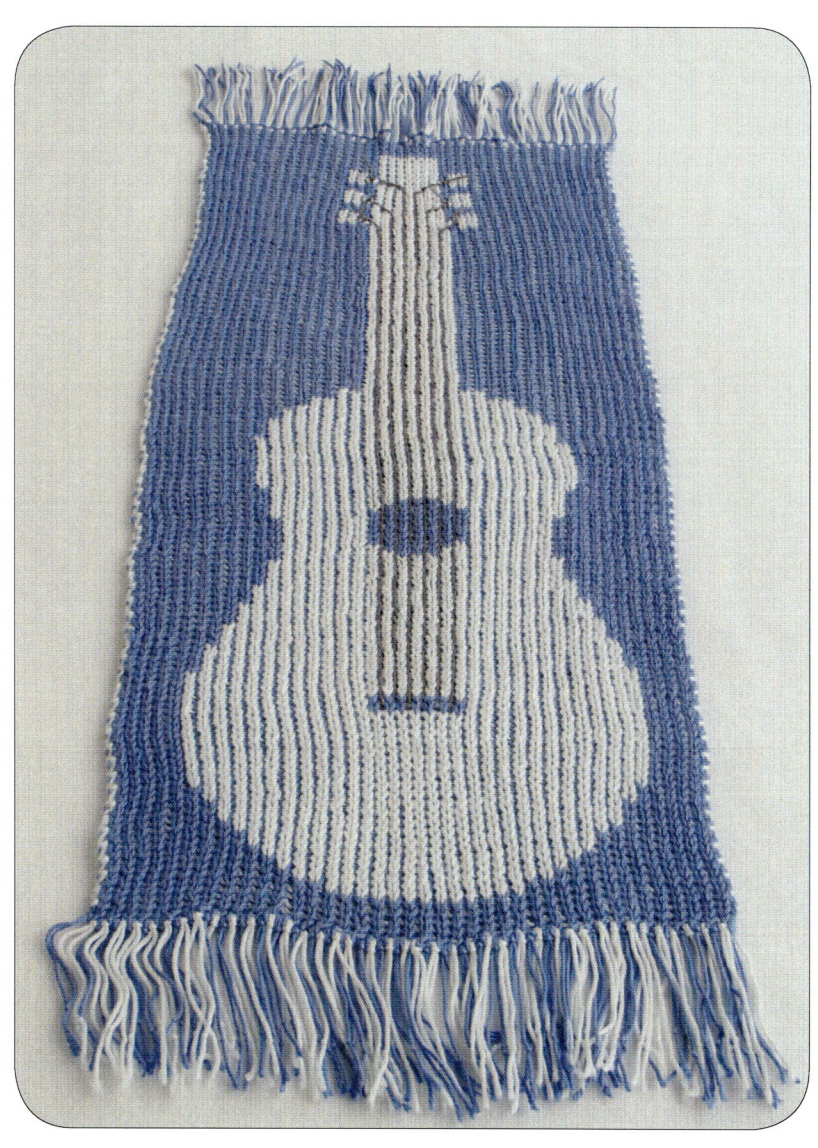

Electric Bass Guitar

An electric bass guitar lends itself to wild and wonderful colors. Use your imagination.
   The four rows of embroidered strings go right up the middle and attach to the knobs at the top.

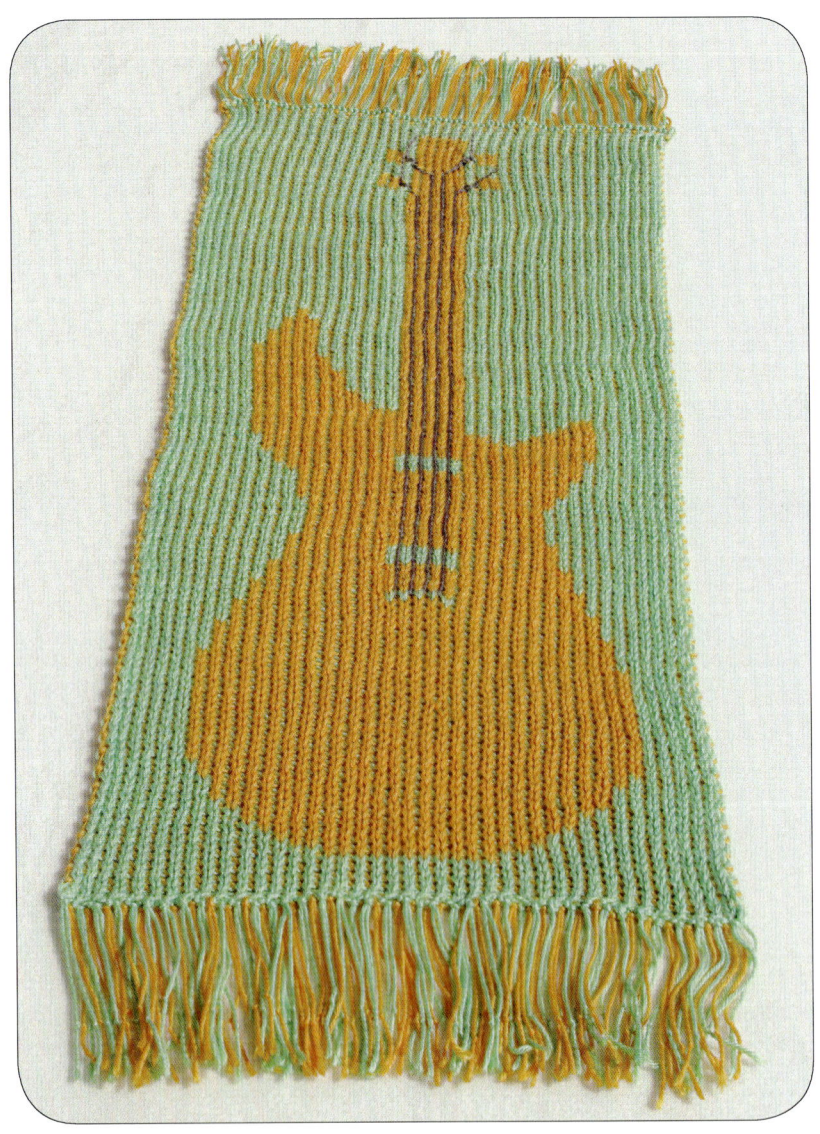

Come Fly with Me

This simple toy airplane has the potential to spark a child's imagination. Where would you fly if you had the chance? Up, up, and away!

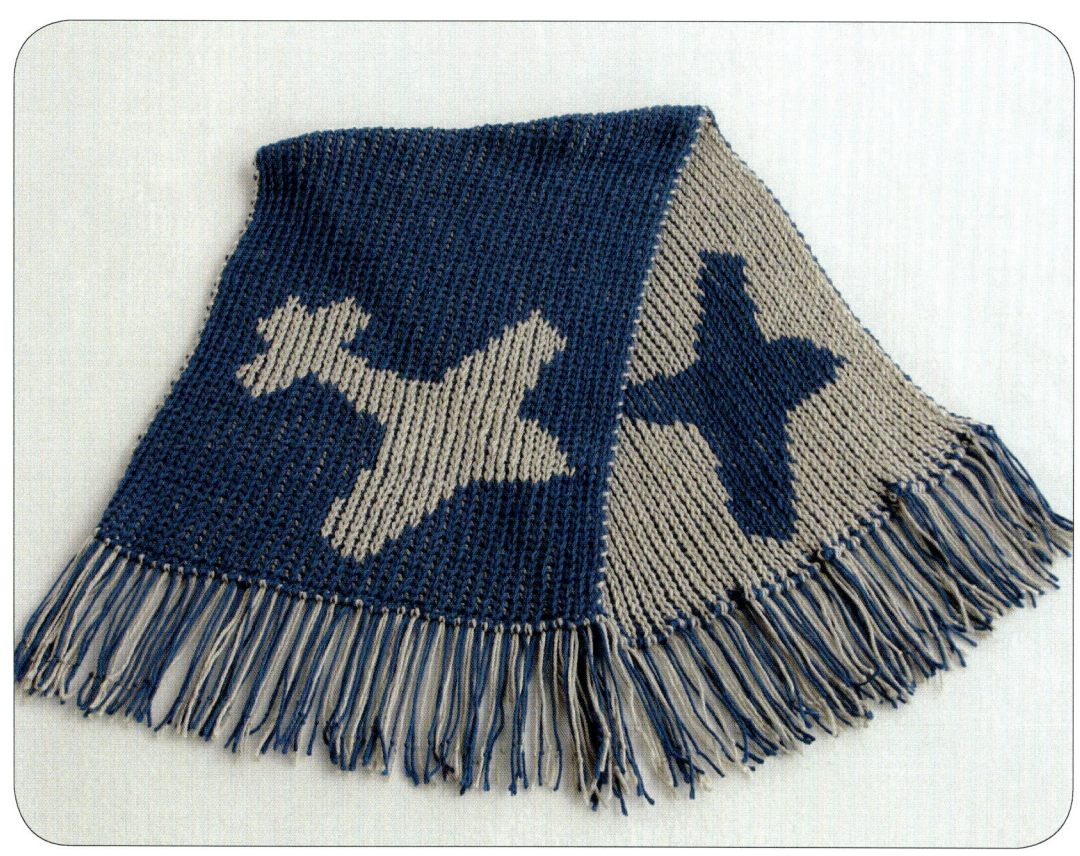

Quiet Sailboats

It is such a peaceful feeling to be quietly sailing over the rolling waves in your very own sailboat. Feel yourself relax as your sailboat rocks you gently in the afternoon breeze.

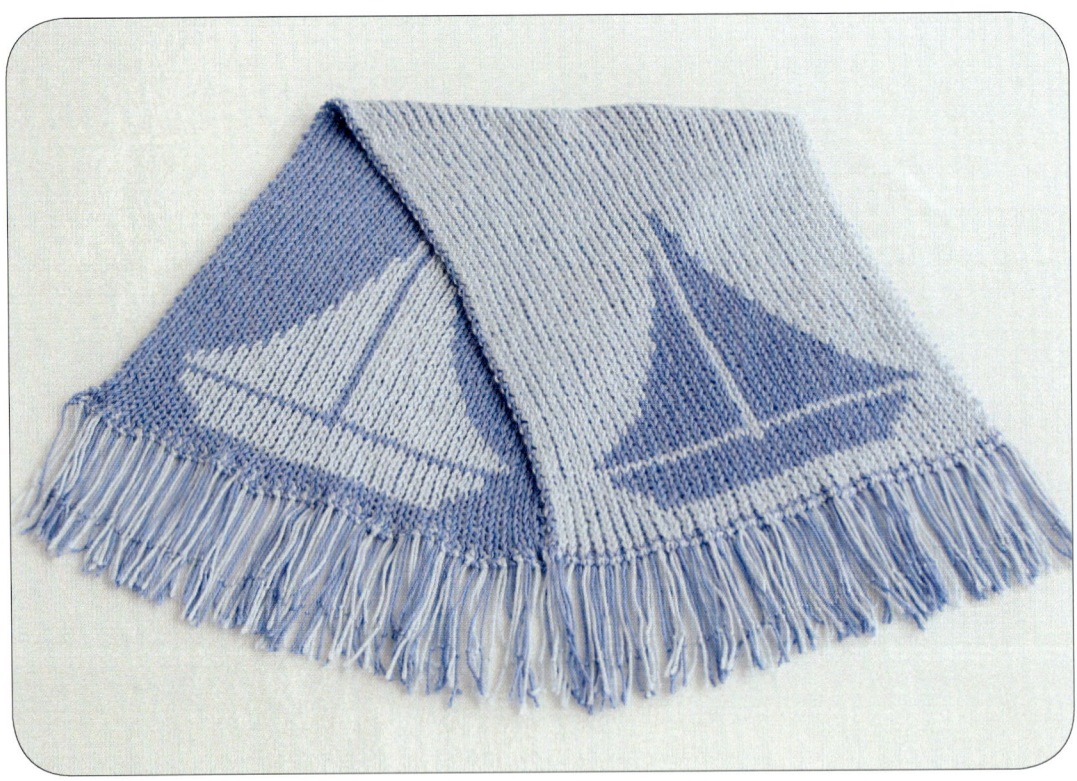

Beautiful Butterflies

These lovely butterflies are just waiting to come to rest on your shoulders. Imagine the limitless number of colors that can be used to create this pattern. Antennae can be added with a chain stitch.

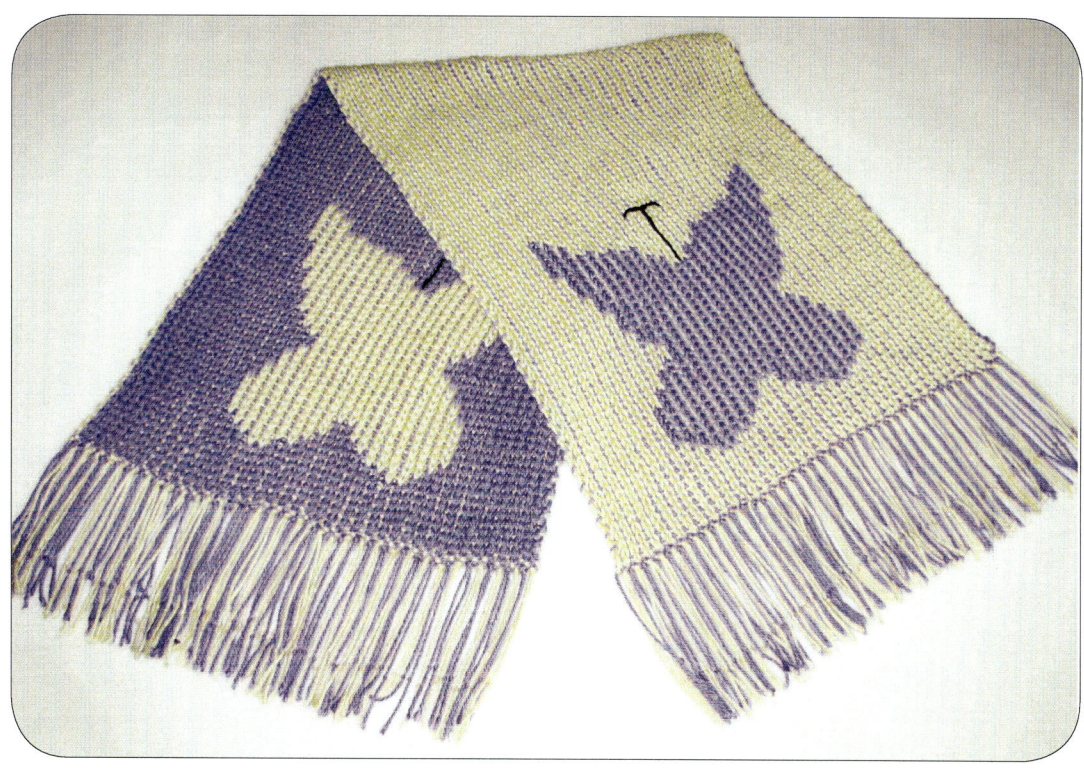

Ducks in a Row

Marching along behind Mother Duck are a row of babies learning to swim, hunt, and just have fun.

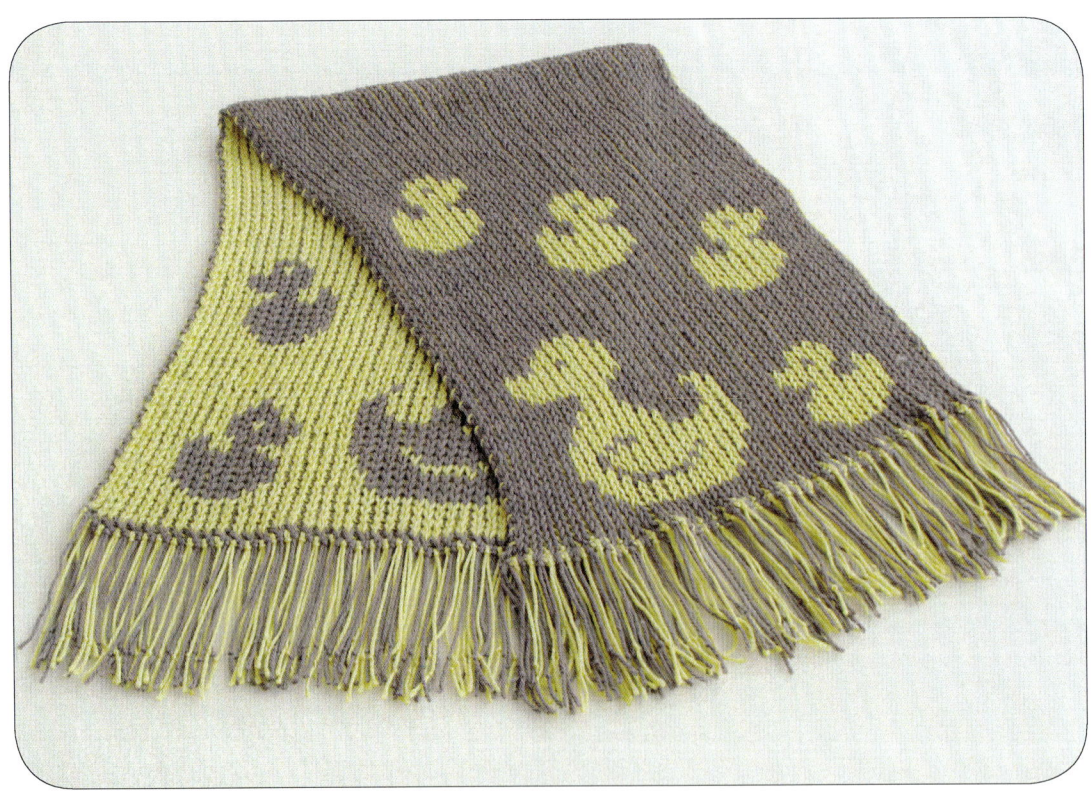

Scottie Dogs

On their leash, these black and white Scotties are ready to go for a walk.

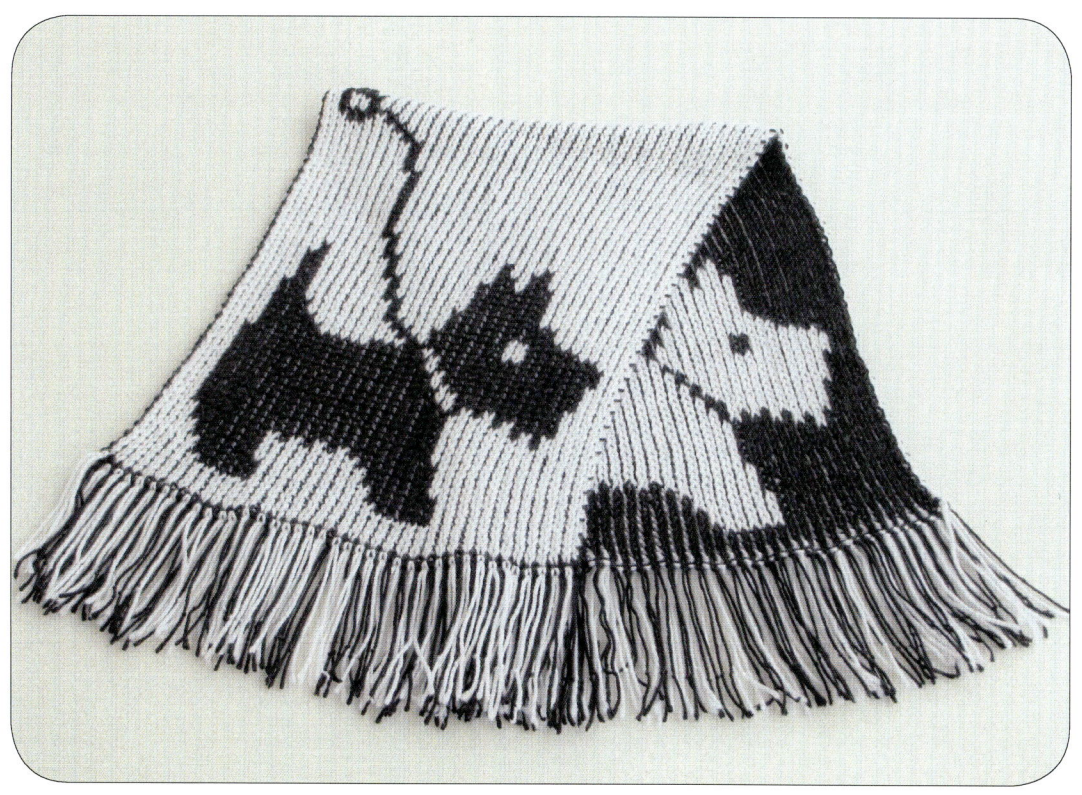

Angels

A child of any age will feel comforted by the serenity of angels wrapped around their shoulders.

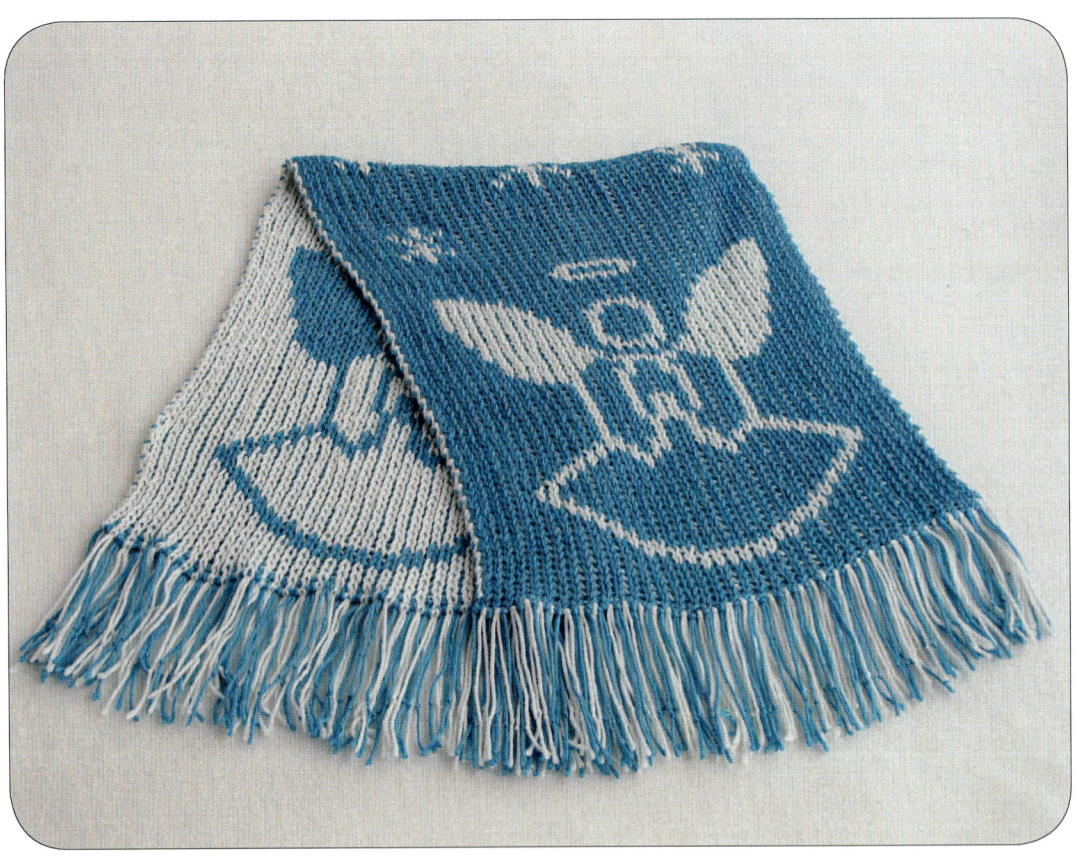

PATTERNS

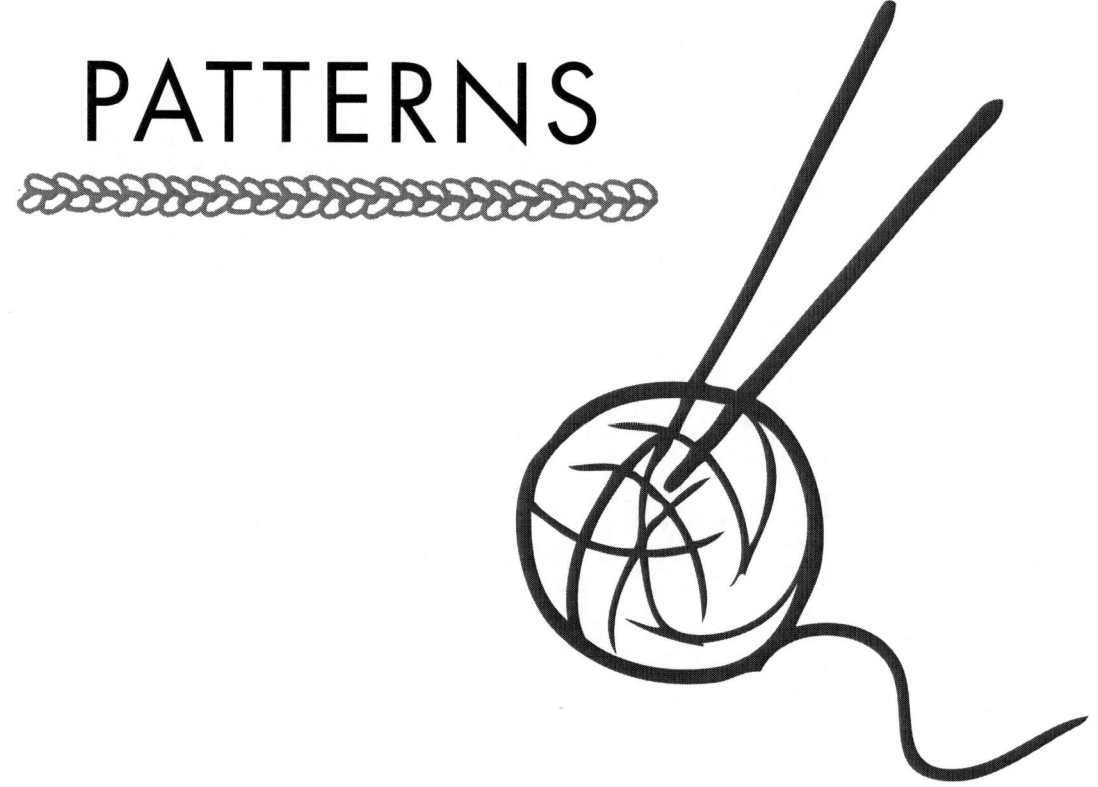

Happy Faces

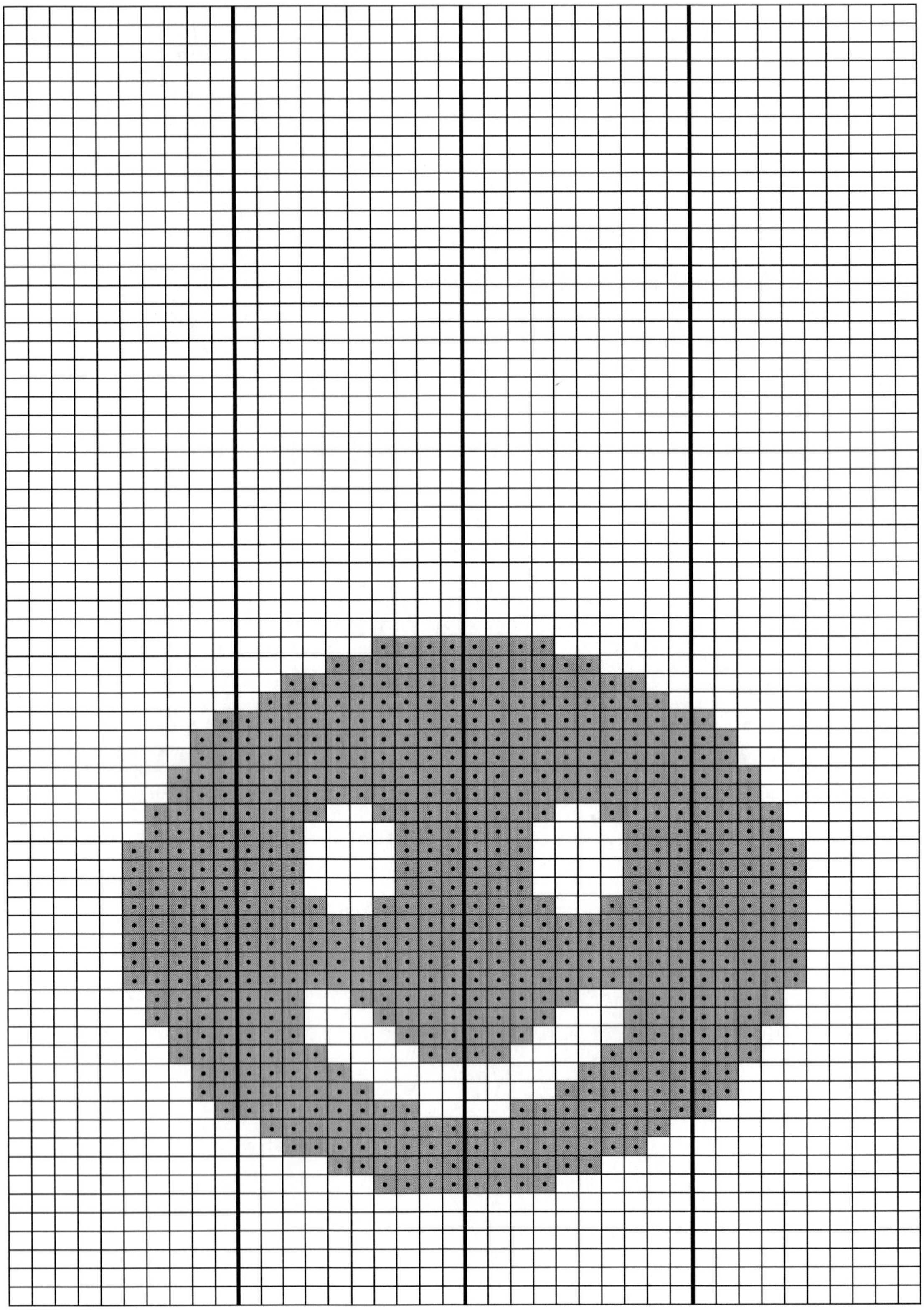

34 SYLVIA SCOTT

Heart Happy Faces

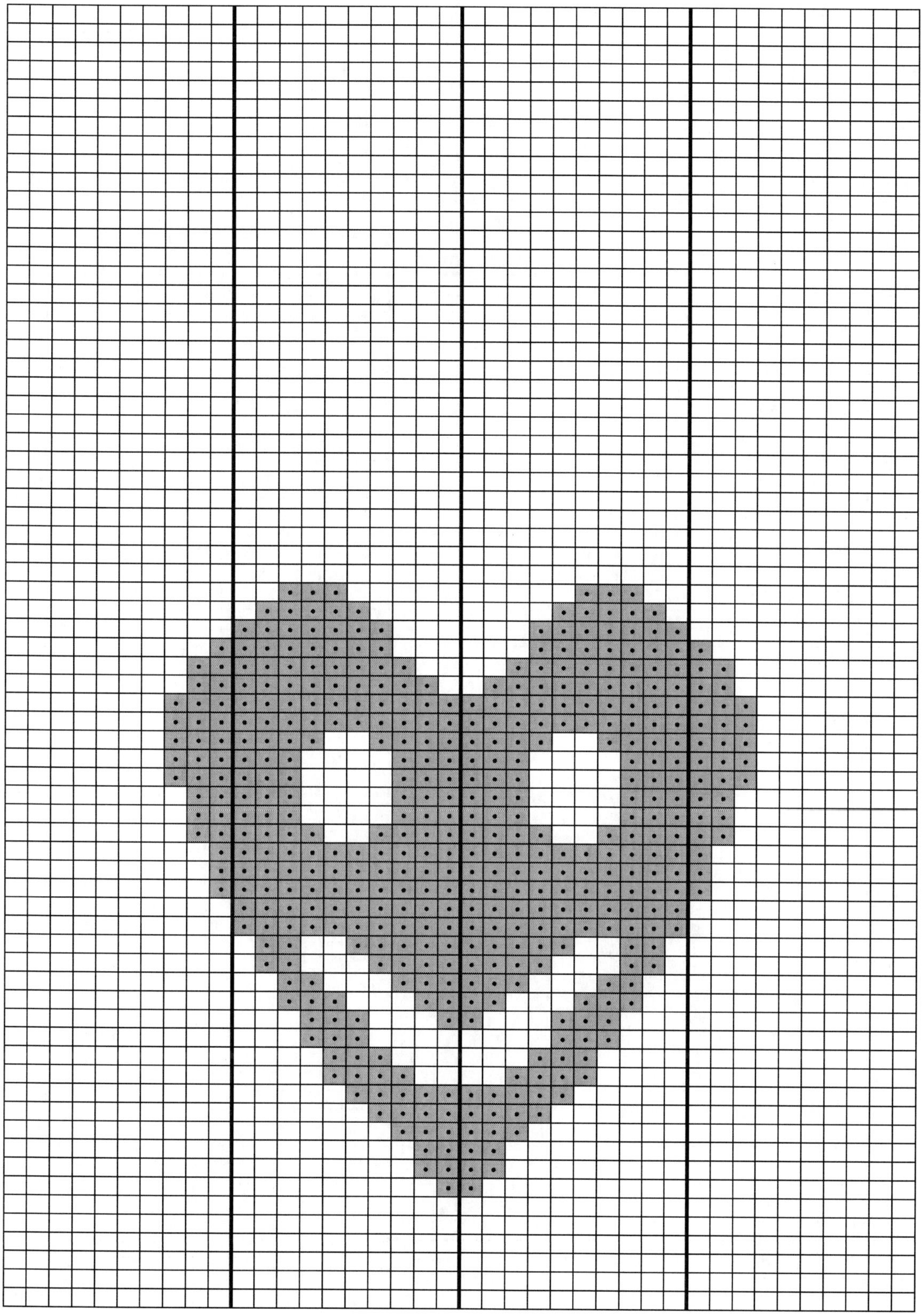

Ascending Hearts

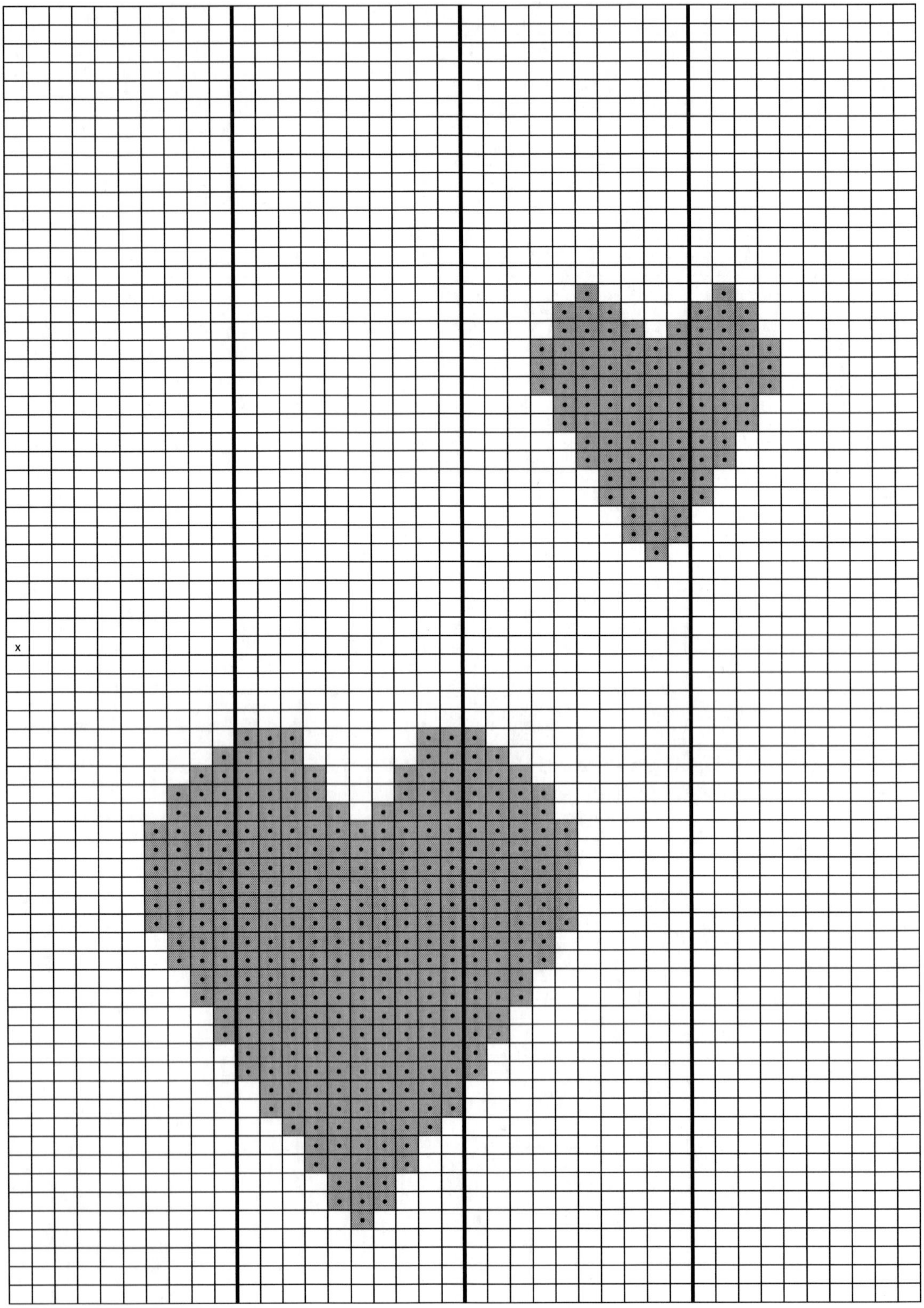

SYLVIA SCOTT

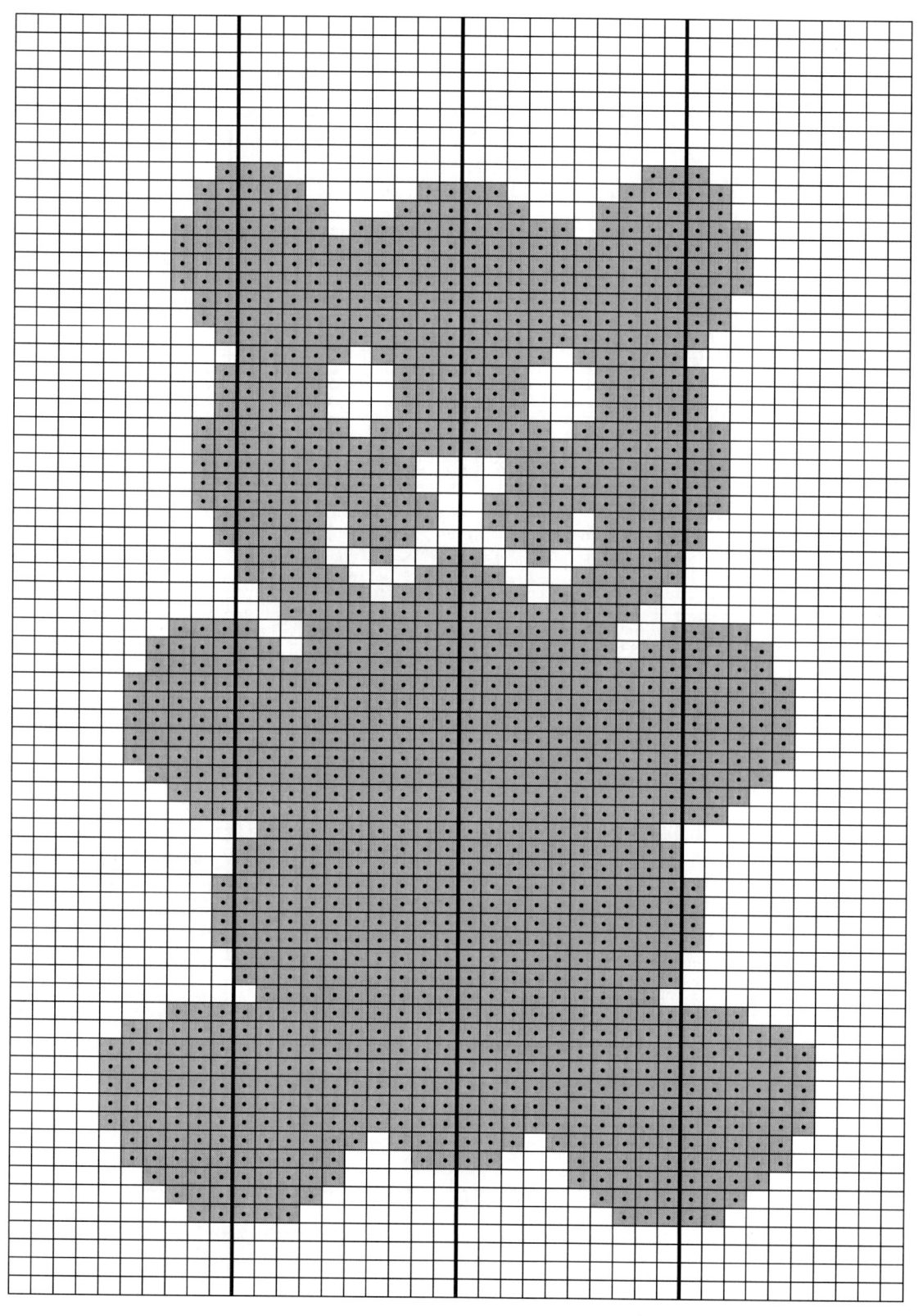

Teddy Bears

WRAPPED IN LOVE

Two Sports Balls

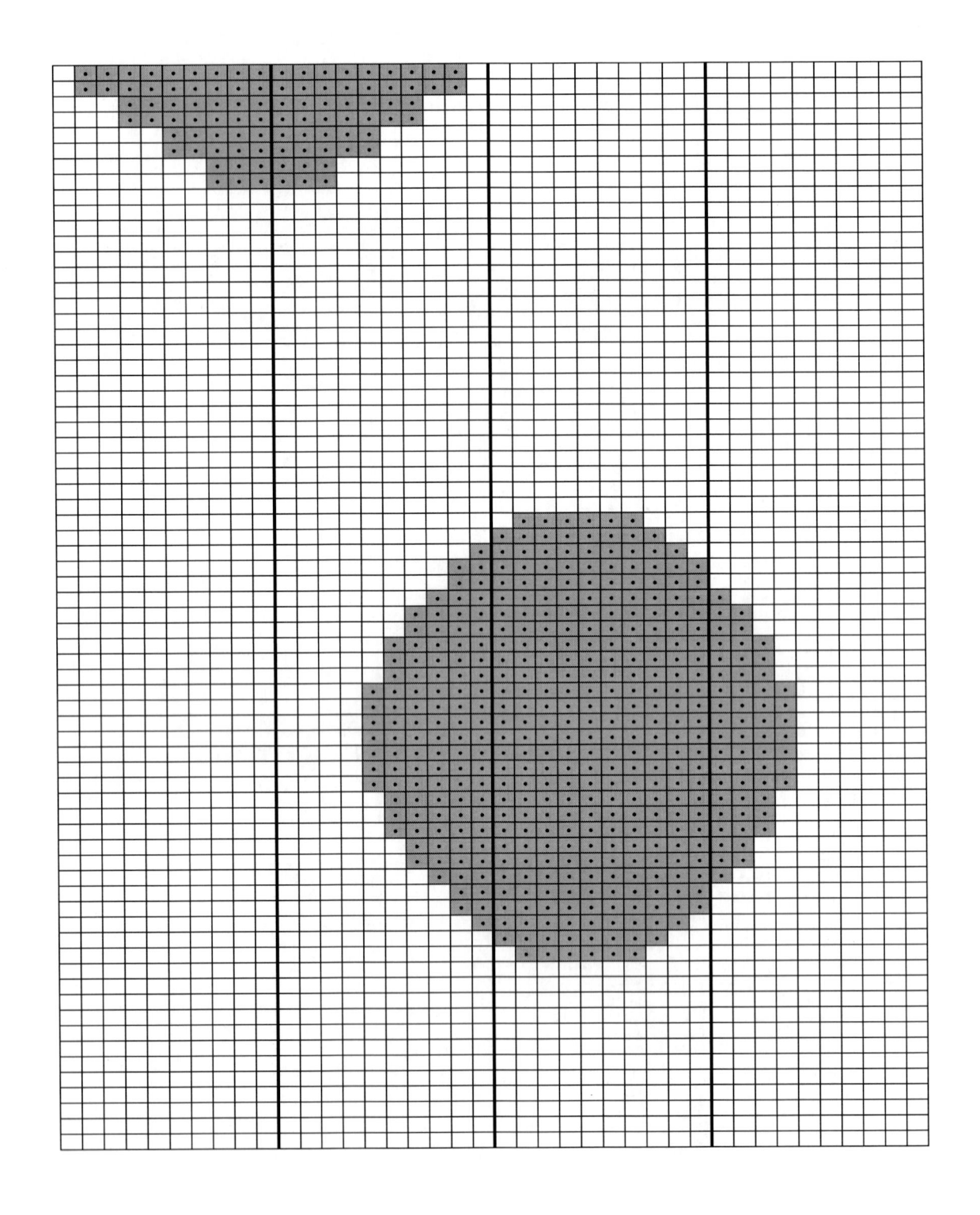

38

SYLVIA SCOTT

Skateboards

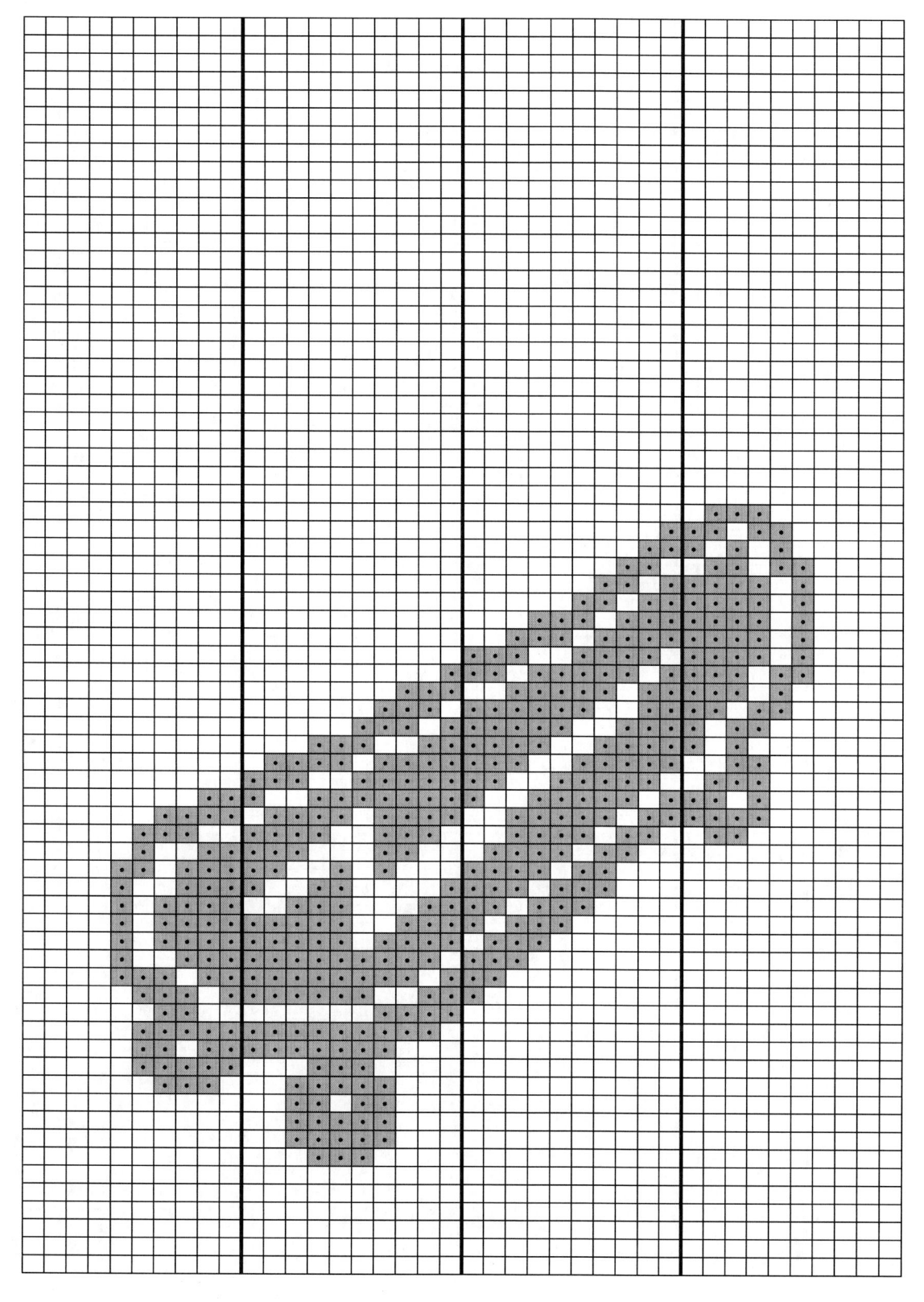

WRAPPED IN LOVE 39

Downhill Bicycles

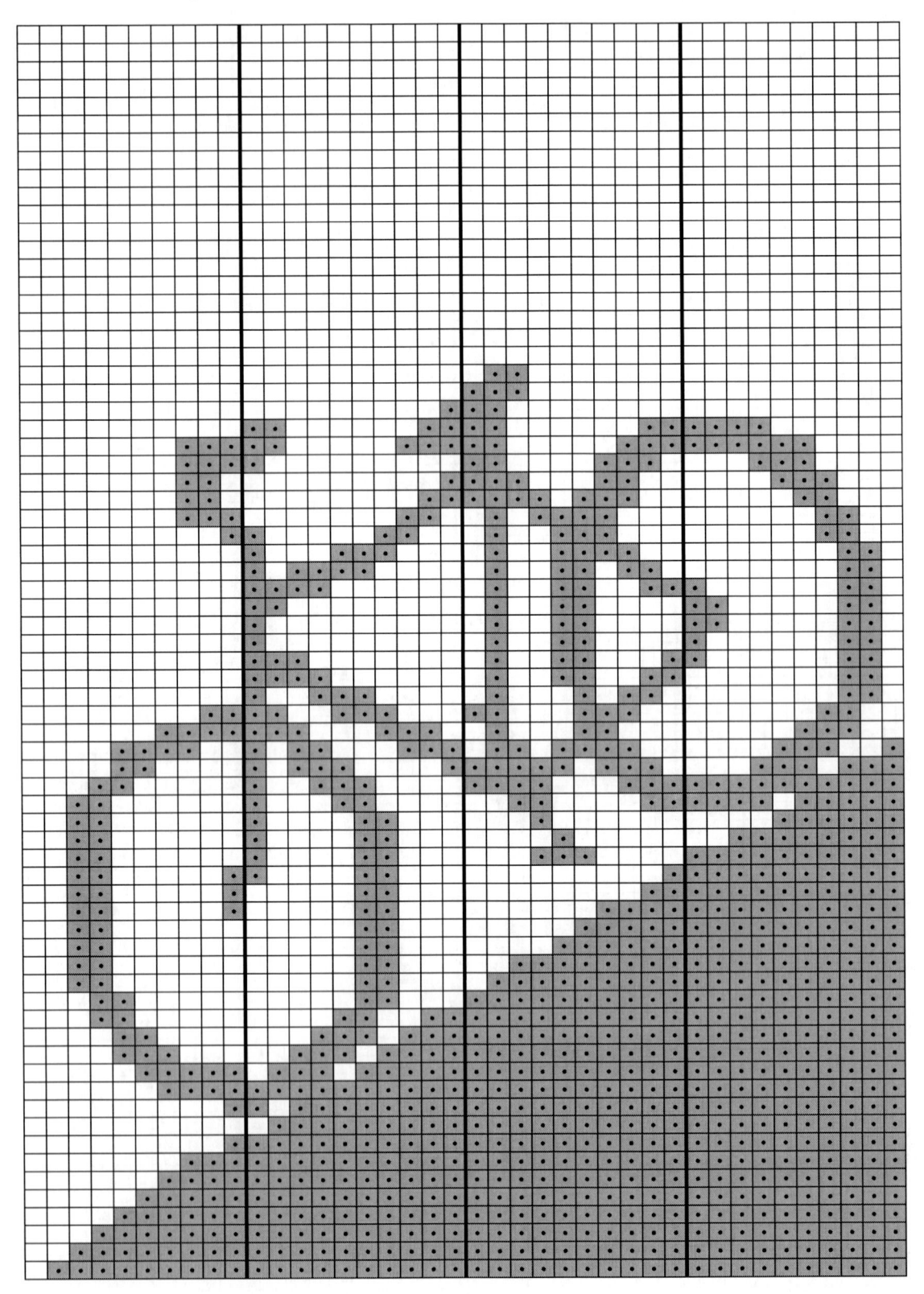

40 SYLVIA SCOTT

Let's Play Football

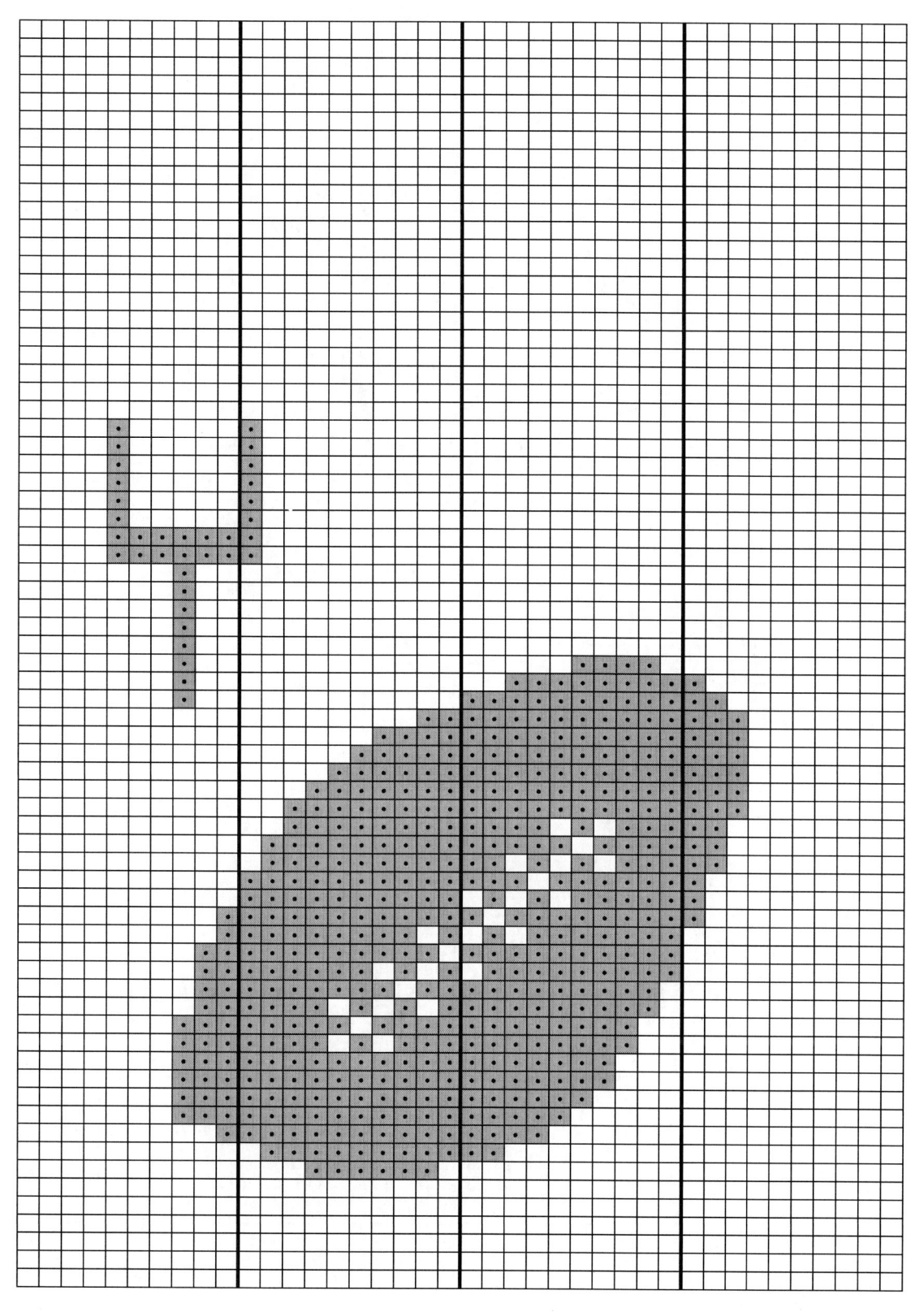

Acoustic Guitar

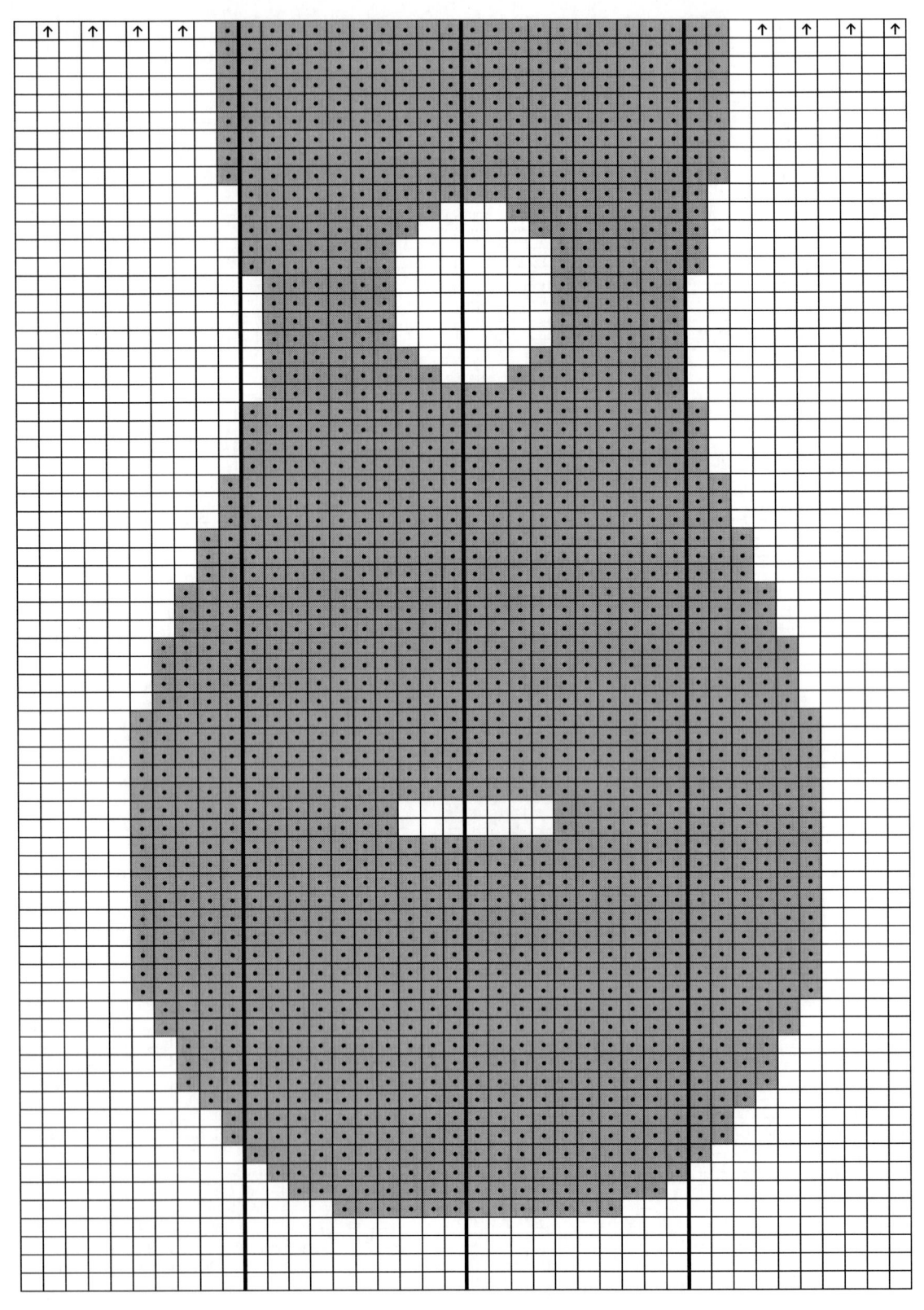

SYLVIA SCOTT

WRAPPED IN LOVE 43

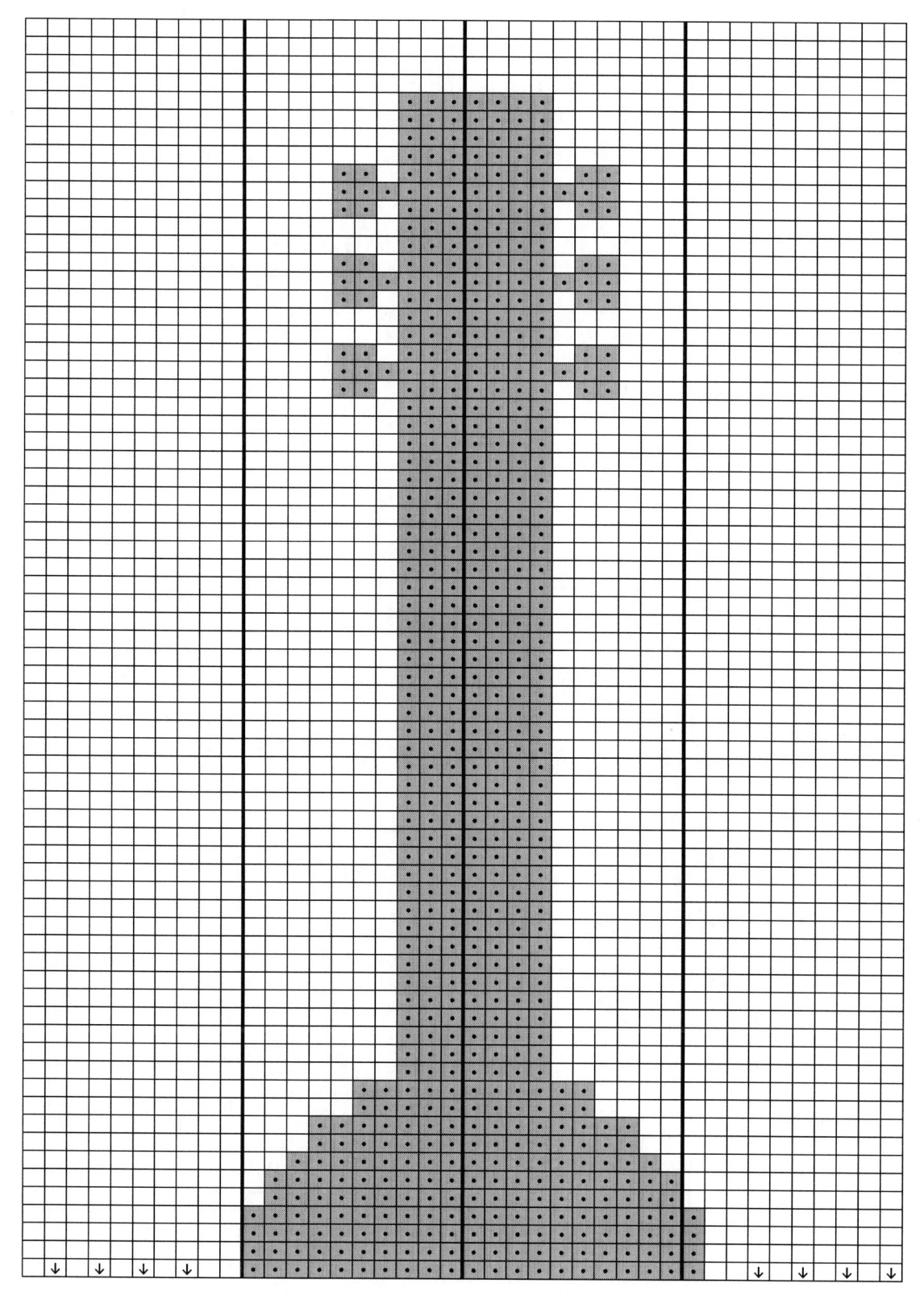

Electric Bass Guitar

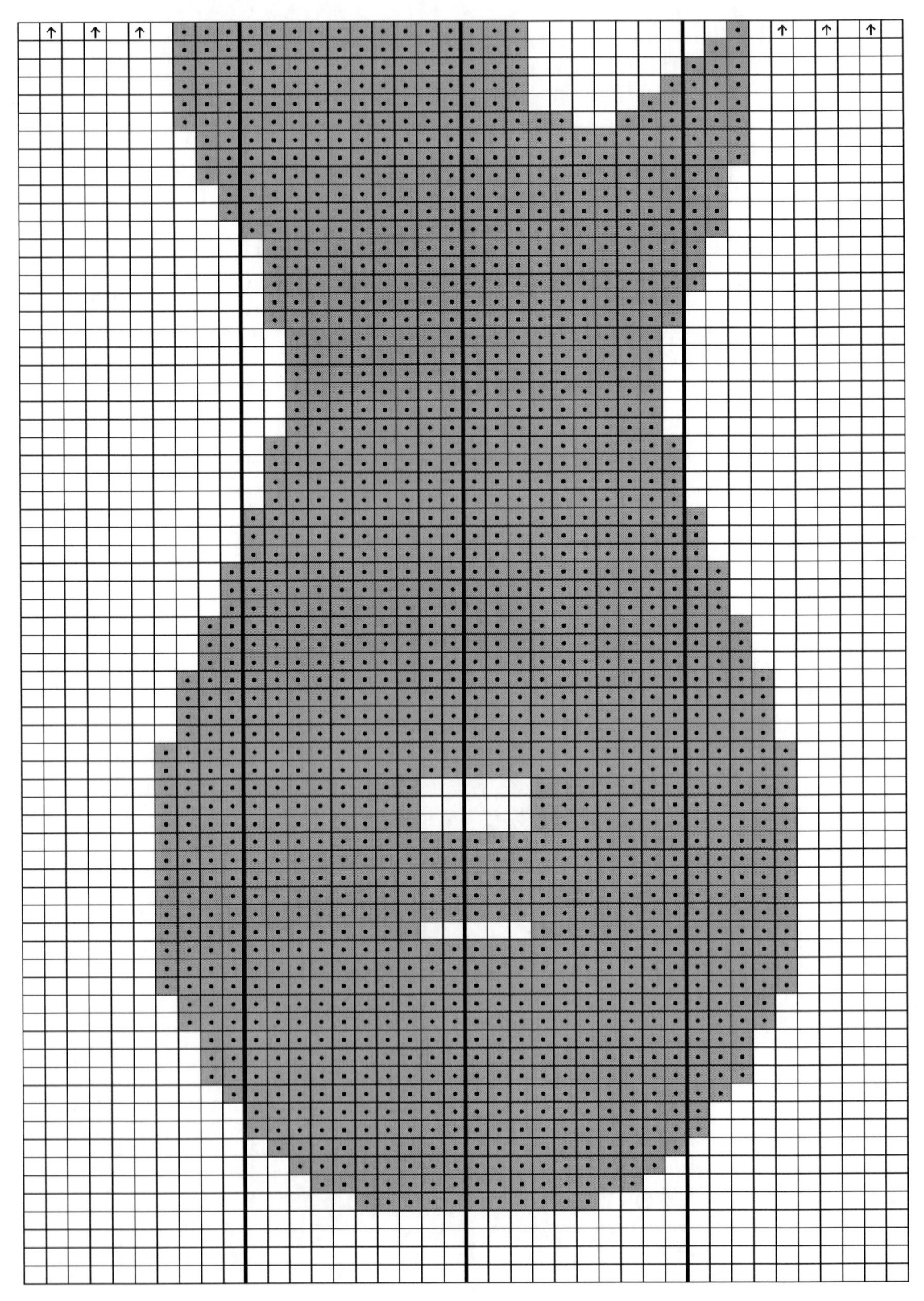

WRAPPED IN LOVE

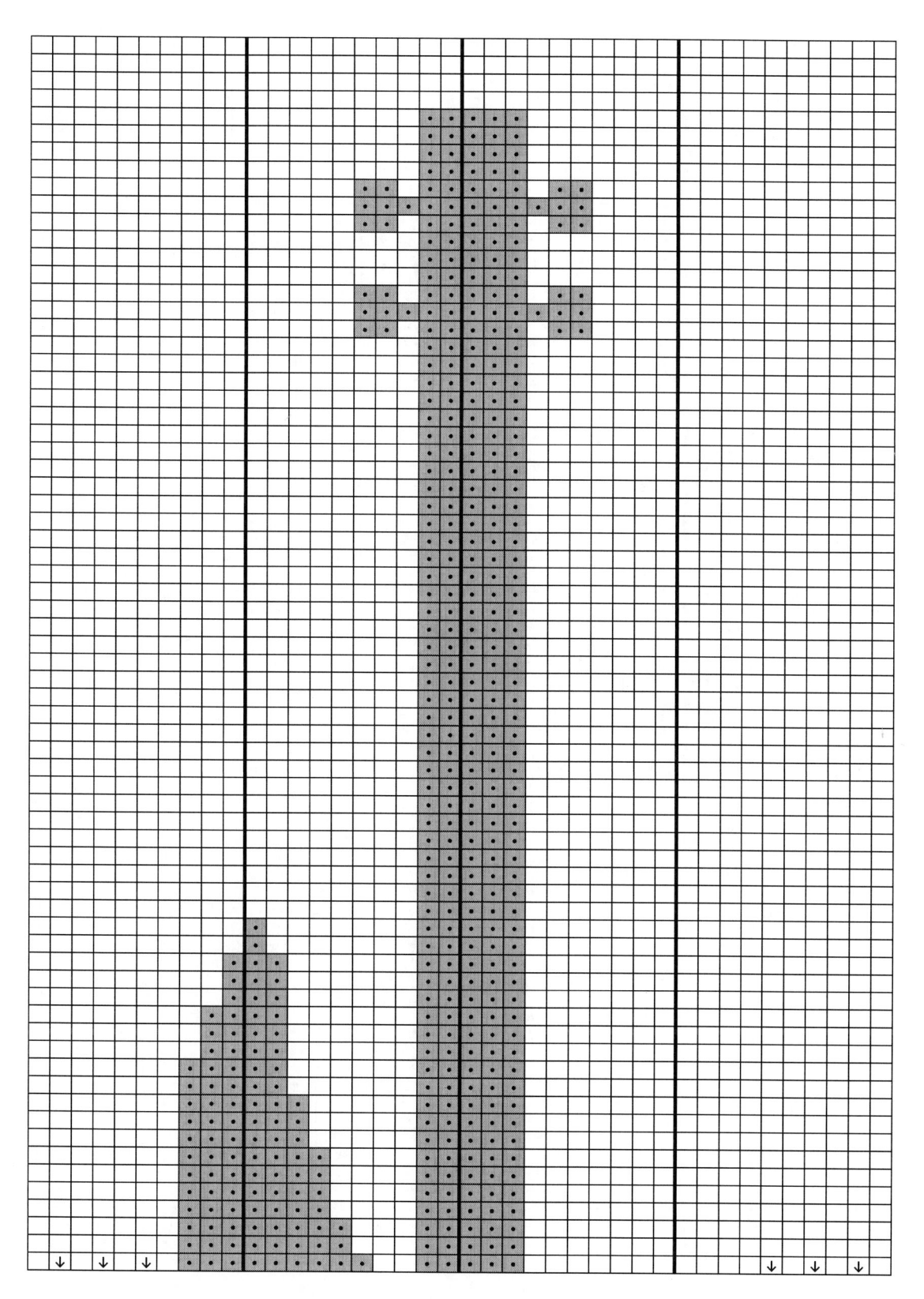

Come Fly with Me

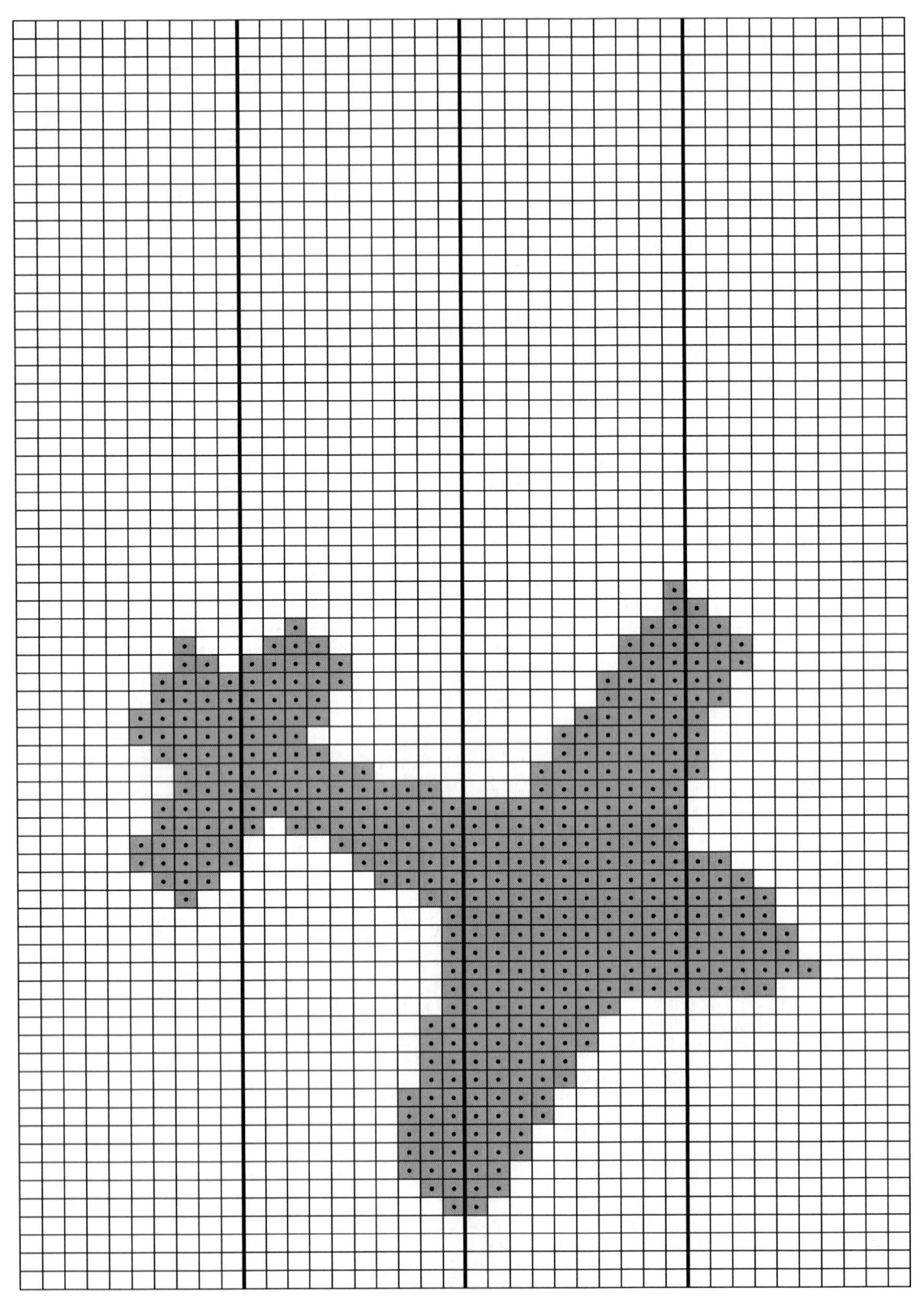

46

SYLVIA SCOTT

Quiet Sailboats

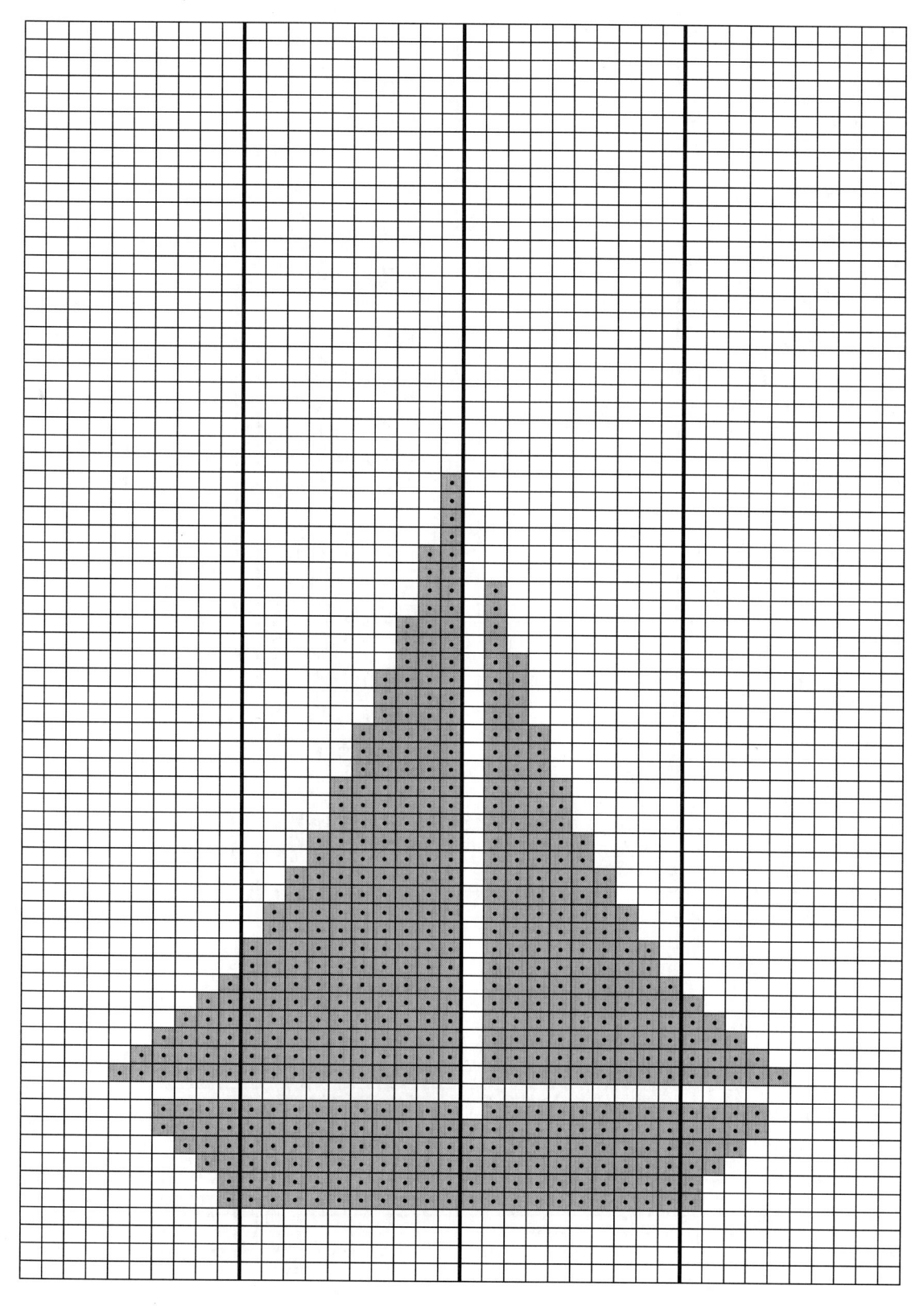

WRAPPED IN LOVE

Beautiful Butterflies

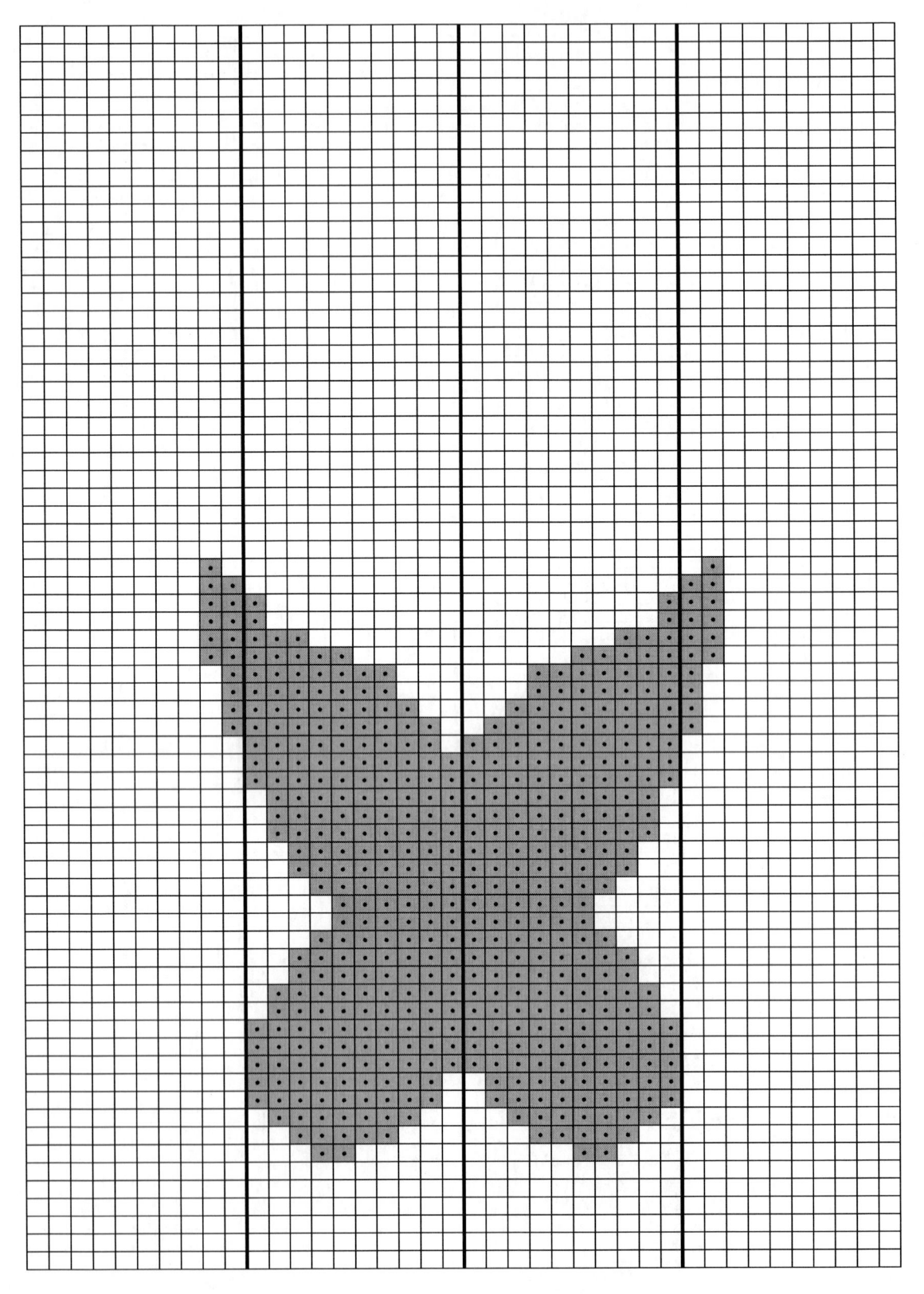

48   SYLVIA SCOTT

Ducks in a Row

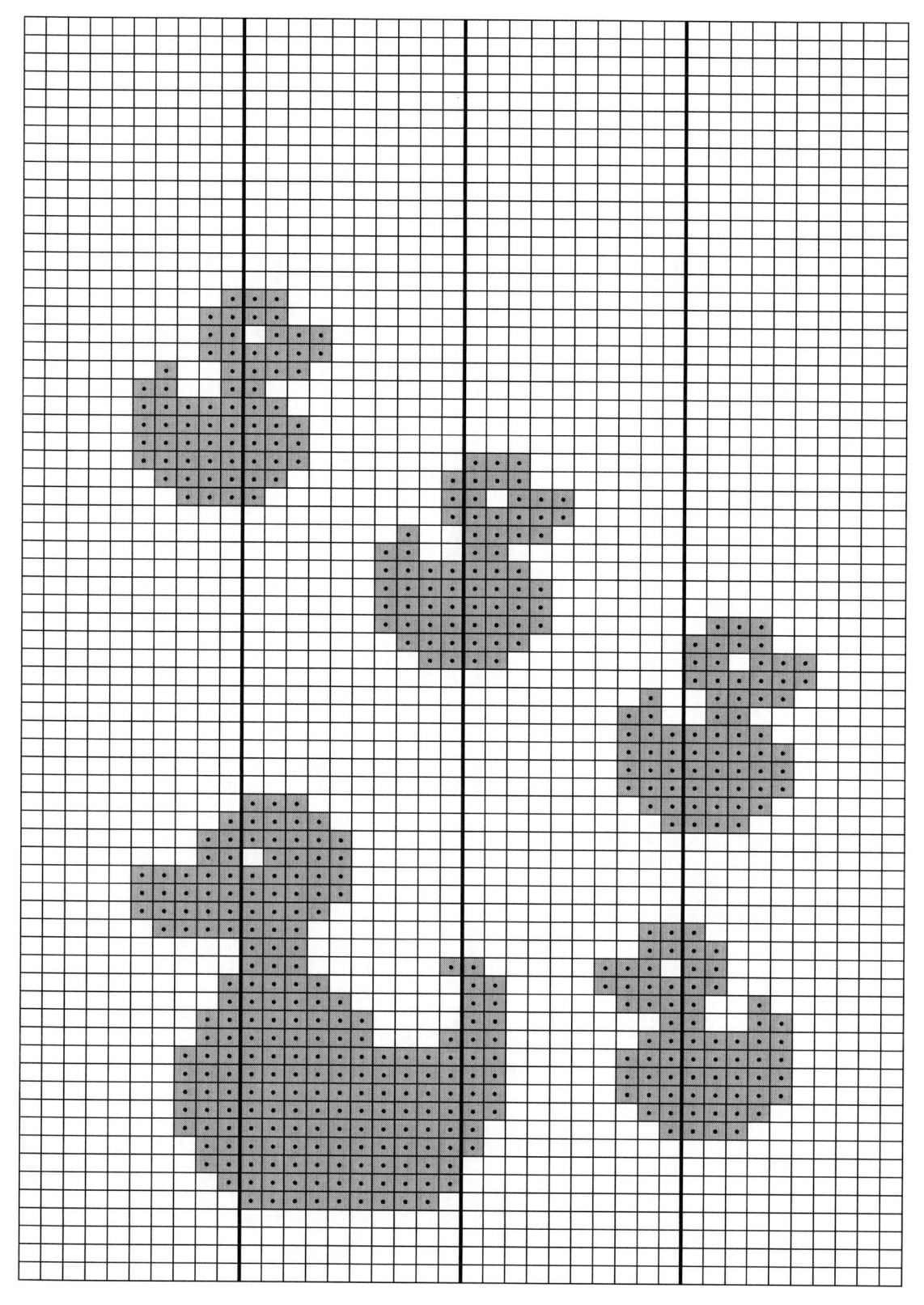

WRAPPED IN LOVE

Scottie Dogs

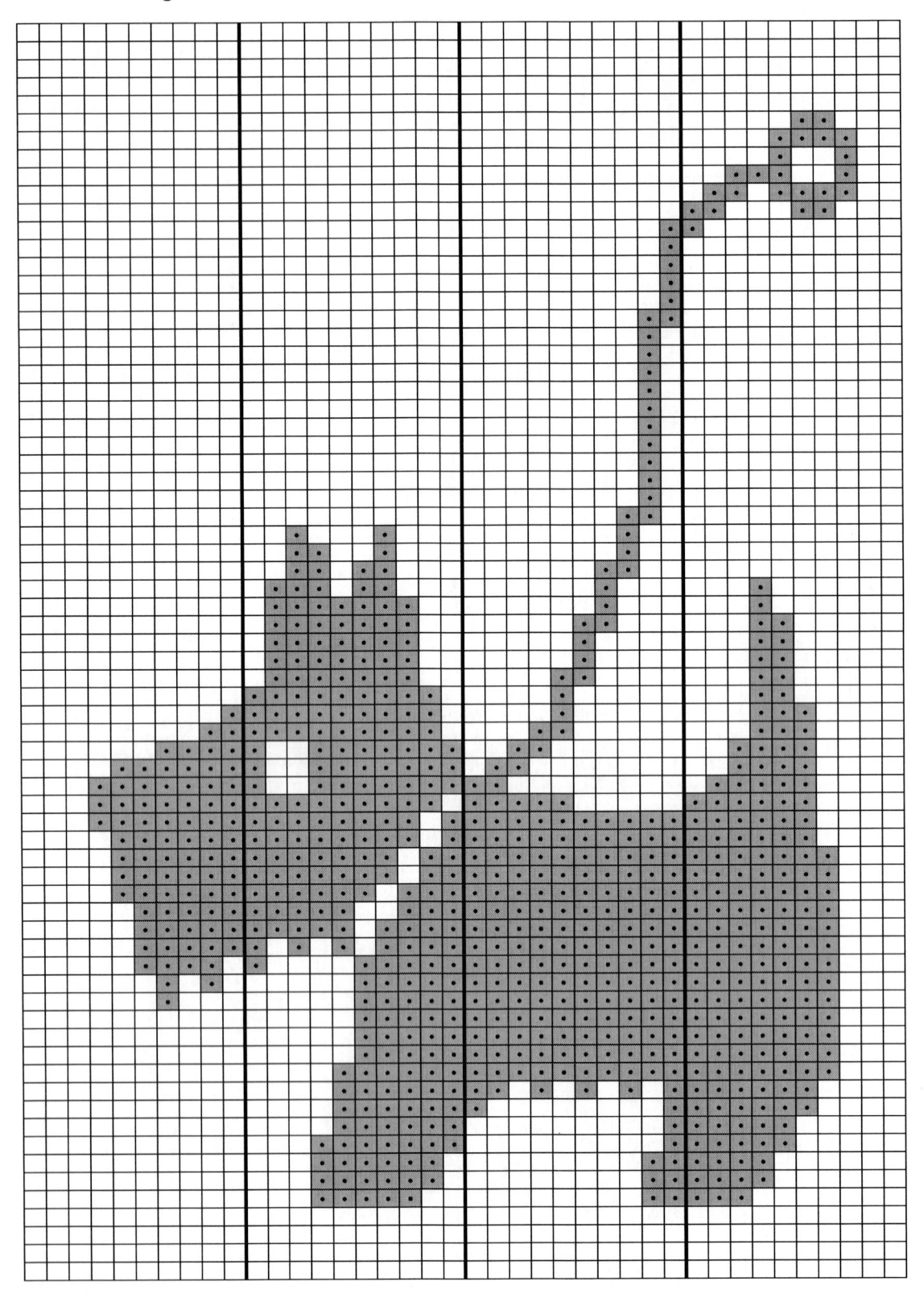

50

SYLVIA SCOTT

Angels

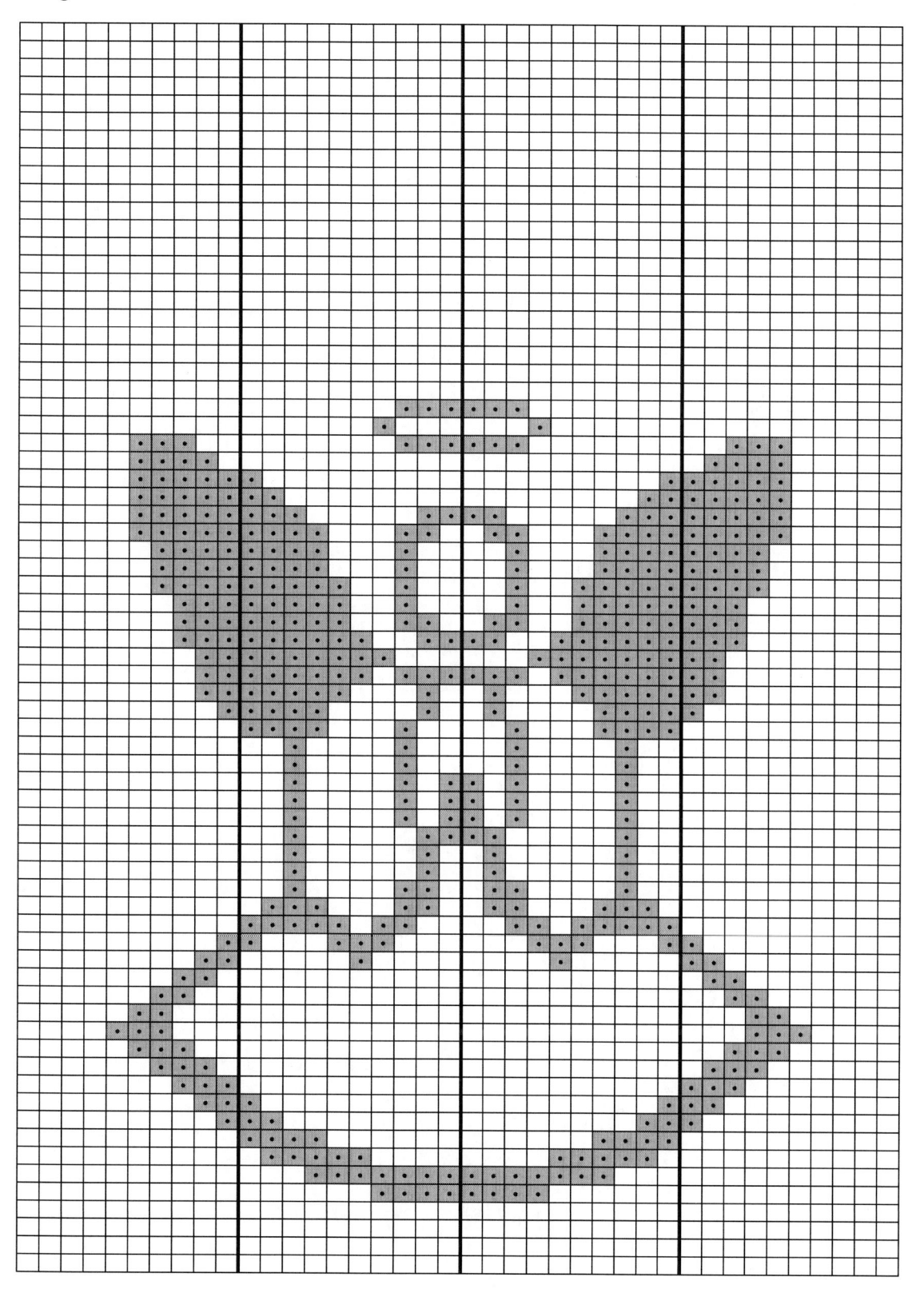

WRAPPED IN LOVE